… NATIONAL ACADEMIES Sciences Engineering Medicine

NATIONAL ACADEMIES PRESS
Washington, DC

Addressing the Needs of an Aging Population Through Health Professions Education

Patricia A. Cuff and
Erin Hammers Forstag, *Rapporteurs*

Global Forum on Innovation in
Health Professional Education

Board on Global Health

Health and Medicine Division

Proceedings of a Workshop

THE NATIONAL ACADEMIES PRESS 500 Fifth Street, NW Washington, DC 20001

This activity was supported by contracts between the National Academy of Sciences and Academic Collaborative for Integrative Health, Academy of Nutrition and Dietetics, Accreditation Council for Graduate Medical Education, American Academy of Nursing, American Association of Colleges of Osteopathic Medicine, American Board of Family Medicine, American Council of Academic Physical Therapy, American Dental Education Association, American Medical Association, American Nurses Credentialing Center, American Occupational Therapy Association, American Physical Therapy Association, American Psychological Association, American Speech-Language-Hearing Association, Association of American Medical Colleges, Association of Schools and Colleges of Optometry, Association of Schools of Advancing Health Professions, Athletic Training Strategic Alliance, Columbia University Vagelos College of Physicians and Surgeons, Council on Social Work Education, the George Washington University, Josiah Macy Jr. Foundation, National Academies of Practice, National Association of Social Workers, National Board for Certified Counselors and Affiliates, National Board of Medical Examiners, National Council of State Boards of Nursing, National League for Nursing, Physician Assistant Education Association, Society for Simulation in Healthcare, Texas A&M University–San Antonio, Texas Tech University Health Sciences Center, U.S. Department of Veterans Affairs, and Weill Cornell Medicine–Qatar. Any opinions, findings, conclusions, or recommendations expressed in this publication do not necessarily reflect the views of any organization or agency that provided support for the project.

International Standard Book Number-13: 978-0-309-70604-9
International Standard Book Number-10: 0-309-70604-1
Digital Object Identifier: https://doi.org/10.17226/27136

This publication is available from the National Academies Press, 500 Fifth Street, NW, Keck 360, Washington, DC 20001; (800) 624-6242 or (202) 334-3313; http://www.nap.edu.

Copyright 2023 by the National Academy of Sciences. National Academies of Sciences, Engineering, and Medicine and National Academies Press and the graphical logos for each are all trademarks of the National Academy of Sciences. All rights reserved.

Printed in the United States of America.

Suggested citation: National Academies of Sciences, Engineering, and Medicine. 2023. *Addressing the needs of an aging population through health professions education: Proceedings of a workshop.* Washington, DC: The National Academies Press. doi: https://doi.org/10.17226/27136.

The **National Academy of Sciences** was established in 1863 by an Act of Congress, signed by President Lincoln, as a private, nongovernmental institution to advise the nation on issues related to science and technology. Members are elected by their peers for outstanding contributions to research. Dr. Marcia McNutt is president.

The **National Academy of Engineering** was established in 1964 under the charter of the National Academy of Sciences to bring the practices of engineering to advising the nation. Members are elected by their peers for extraordinary contributions to engineering. Dr. John L. Anderson is president.

The **National Academy of Medicine** (formerly the Institute of Medicine) was established in 1970 under the charter of the National Academy of Sciences to advise the nation on medical and health issues. Members are elected by their peers for distinguished contributions to medicine and health. Dr. Victor J. Dzau is president.

The three Academies work together as the **National Academies of Sciences, Engineering, and Medicine** to provide independent, objective analysis and advice to the nation and conduct other activities to solve complex problems and inform public policy decisions. The National Academies also encourage education and research, recognize outstanding contributions to knowledge, and increase public understanding in matters of science, engineering, and medicine.

Learn more about the National Academies of Sciences, Engineering, and Medicine at **www.nationalacademies.org**.

Consensus Study Reports published by the National Academies of Sciences, Engineering, and Medicine document the evidence-based consensus on the study's statement of task by an authoring committee of experts. Reports typically include findings, conclusions, and recommendations based on information gathered by the committee and the committee's deliberations. Each report has been subjected to a rigorous and independent peer-review process and it represents the position of the National Academies on the statement of task.

Proceedings published by the National Academies of Sciences, Engineering, and Medicine chronicle the presentations and discussions at a workshop, symposium, or other event convened by the National Academies. The statements and opinions contained in proceedings are those of the participants and are not endorsed by other participants, the planning committee, or the National Academies.

Rapid Expert Consultations published by the National Academies of Sciences, Engineering, and Medicine are authored by subject-matter experts on narrowly focused topics that can be supported by a body of evidence. The discussions contained in rapid expert consultations are considered those of the authors and do not contain policy recommendations. Rapid expert consultations are reviewed by the institution before release.

For information about other products and activities of the National Academies, please visit www.nationalacademies.org/about/whatwedo.

PLANNING COMMITTEE ON ADDRESSING THE NEEDS OF AN AGING POPULATION THROUGH HEALTH PROFESSIONS EDUCATION[1]

DONNA FERGUSON (*Cochair*), Department of Defense
ANDREA PFEIFLE (*Cochair*), National Academies of Practice
NICOLE ANSELME, Strategic Healthcare Programs LLC
RICARDO CUSTODIO, University of Hawaii West O'ahu
ELIZABETH GOLDBLATT, Strategic Healthcare Programs, LLC
GREG HARTLEY, University of Miami
JENNIFER KIM, Vanderbilt University School of Nursing
KATHRYN KOLASA, Brody School of Medicine, East Carolina University
CATHY MAXWELL, Vanderbilt University School of Nursing
LAUREN MAZZURCO, Eastern Virginia Medical School
SENTHIL RAJASEKARAN, Khalifa University College of Medicine and Health Sciences
JOANNE SCHWARTZBERG, American Medical Association
ZOHRAY TALIB, California University of Science and Medicine

Learners and Consultants to the Planning Committee
RIHAM ABU AFFAN, Khalifa University
LILY BRICKMAN, University of Maine
DARLA SPENCE COFFEY, Council on Social Work Education
REBECCA GEORGE, University of California Davis
BROOKE HAZEN, Vanderbilt University School of Nursing
CHERYL HOYING, National League for Nursing

---

[1] The National Academies of Sciences, Engineering, and Medicine's forums and roundtables do not issue, review, or approve individual documents. The responsibility for the published Proceedings of a Workshop rests with the workshop rapporteurs and the institution.

Reviewers

This Proceedings of a Workshop was reviewed in draft form by individuals chosen for their diverse perspectives and technical expertise. The purpose of this independent review is to provide candid and critical comments that will assist the National Academies of Sciences, Engineering, and Medicine in making each published proceedings as sound as possible and to ensure that it meets the institutional standards for quality, objectivity, evidence, and responsiveness to the charge. The review comments and draft manuscript remain confidential to protect the integrity of the process.

We thank the following individuals for their review of this proceedings:

CATHY A. MAXWELL, Vanderbilt University
DARLA SPENCE COFFEY, (Rtd) Council on Social Work Education

Although the reviewers listed above provided many constructive comments and suggestions, they were not asked to endorse the content of the proceedings nor did they see the final draft before its release. The review of this proceedings was overseen by **DEBORAH E. POWELL,** University of Minnesota. She was responsible for making certain that an independent examination of this proceedings was carried out in accordance with standards of the National Academies and that all review comments were carefully considered. Responsibility for the final content rests entirely with the rapporteurs and the National Academies.

Contents

1	Introduction and Framing of the Issues	1
2	Exploring What Matters Most in Working with Older Adults	17
3	Supply and Demand: Is the Workforce Prepared to Meet the Needs of Older Adults?	29
4	Addressing the Gap	41
5	Making It Happen with Implementation Science	57

APPENDIXES

A	References	69
B	Members of the Global Forum on Innovation in Health Professional Education	73
C	Workshop Agenda	81
D	Planning Committee and Speaker Biographies	87

1

Introduction[1] and Framing of the Issues

The Global Forum on Innovation in Health Professional Education[2] at the National Academies of Sciences, Engineering, and Medicine held a workshop on Addressing the Needs of an Aging Population through Health Professions Education on December 7–8, 2022. A pre-workshop session took place on November 15, 2022, to introduce the topic through an implementation science lens. Although there was an option to attend the workshop in person in Washington, D.C., participants primarily joined virtually. The workshop and pre-workshop agendas were planned by an expert planning committee (see Appendix D) whose work was guided by a Statement of Task (Box 1-1).

Of note is that these proceedings are organized by subject area, rather than chronologically (see Agenda in Appendix C). Chapter 1 opens with a framing discussion focused on the perspectives and needs of patients. This brief introduction is followed by presentations and discussions about working with older adults, learner reluctance to work with older adults, and speakers' views on applying the World Health Organization's intrinsic capacity framework within and across health professions. Chapter 2 presents discussions about educating learners on aging across the life course and

---

[1] The planning committee's role was limited to planning the workshop, and this Proceedings of a Workshop was prepared by the rapporteurs as a factual account of what occurred at the workshop. Statements, recommendations, and opinions expressed are those of individual presenters and participants and are not necessarily endorsed or verified by the National Academies of Sciences, Engineering, and Medicine. They should not be construed as reflecting any group consensus.

[2] See Appendix B for a full list of forum members and staff.

> **BOX 1-1**
> **Statement of Task**
>
> A planning committee of the National Academies of Sciences, Engineering, and Medicine will organize and conduct a public workshop to explore the many and varied needs of an aging population and an ideal health workforce that could match those identified population needs in terms of numbers and skillset. Further discussion will include expert opinions on who will make up the health workforce, training requirements for each level of care provider, who will provide the training and education, and in what setting the training will take place. Learning from global examples can shed light on new ways of addressing shared challenges with aging such as mental health functioning, physical functioning, persistent pain, multi-morbidity, and polypharmacy. How social determinants of health impact a healthy aging process and payment structures to care for a growing older population are equally important areas to consider.
>
> The planning committee will select and invite speakers and discussants and moderate the discussions at the workshop. Following the workshop, a proceedings of the presentations and discussions will be prepared by a designated rapporteur in accordance with institutional guidelines.

summarizes a presentation on an age-friendly health education tool. Chapter 3 explores the question of whether the current health workforce supply is adequate to meet the needs of an aging population. Chapter 4 explores ways to address the gap between supply and demand, with summaries of presentations on a variety of approaches currently in use. Chapter 5 closes the proceedings with a description of implementation science and how it can help health professions education develop evidence-based approaches for building a workforce that is eager and prepared to work with older adults.

FRAMING THE ISSUES

Key Messages from the Presenters[3]

- Health professions education programs do not require classes in geriatrics, and it can be difficult to get programs to even offer elective opportunities to gain experience in geriatric care. (Pfeifle)

---

[3] This list is the rapporteurs' summary of points made by individual speakers, and the statements have not been endorsed or verified by the National Academies of Sciences, Engineering, and Medicine. They are not intended to reflect a consensus among workshop participants.

- Giving older adults the opportunity to be engaged in the community and to help other people is an essential part of healthy aging. (Newton)
- The "elephant in the room" is the need for a paradigm shift in how students are taught to think about older adults and the ideas that shape our attitudes. (Maxwell)
- At the learner level, it is important to move students into the community and learn from older adults directly. (Talib)

Andrea Pfeifle, the associate vice president for interprofessional practice and education for The Ohio State University and Wexner Medical Center, and Donna Ferguson, the mental health and wellness program manager at the Department of the Army Criminal Investigations Command in the Department of Defense, welcomed participants to the workshop by highlighting the importance of building the health care workforce to be prepared to care for the needs of older adults. An implementation science lens, Pfeifle said, is a useful approach for discussing how to make the necessary changes in health professions education. She noted that most health professions education programs do not require classes in geriatrics and said that it can be difficult to get these health professions education programs to even offer elective opportunities for students to gain experience in geriatric care.

The December 7 workshop session began with a conversation among Pfeifle, Ferguson, and community members Nancy Cruz and Willie Ann Burroughs. Pfeifle said that when exploring ways to inspire learners to pursue training and education in the care of older adults, it is critical to keep the focus on the "captain of the ship"—that is, on the older adults themselves who are in a position to make their own life decisions. Ferguson added that a team-based approach is important in both education and care and that the center of the team is the patient. Ferguson asked Cruz and Burroughs to tell workshop participants about themselves, their lives, and their work.

Cruz lives in Queens, New York. After a career working as a nurse in both a hospital and in a school, she now volunteers at the local senior center. She takes seniors' blood pressure readings and listens to their problems; she added that some seniors at the center are "so lonely" and that just being there to listen is "such a big deal for them." Cruz said that at mealtime some of the seniors want to maintain their independence and "eat what they want to eat." She coaches them to try new things but also understands that every once in a while they need a special treat of something they are not supposed to have, "even if the doctor doesn't like it." Cruz said she gets around mostly on foot and is able to walk to the supermarket and many other stores. There are plenty of buses available if she needs to travel farther, such as to the doctor. As a former nurse, Cruz said she is able to communicate easily with her doctors and understand their lingo, but some of the seniors whom she helps cannot. Cruz encourages the seniors to speak up and ask their doctors for what they need. In offering some observations about the health care system in general, Cruz said that most nurses today do not have the time with patients that she had when she was a young nurse; nurses are overwhelmed with 10 to 15 patients and are likely to miss signs and symptoms that are important. Young nurses need support from older nurses and more time with patients, she said; without this support, the system loses many good nurses.

Burroughs lives in Thomasville, Alabama. She drives herself to doctor appointments in Mobile and to visit her children in Birmingham, Mobile, and other places. She helps to care for two "young ladies"; one is 86 years old, and the other is 101 years old. Burroughs helps them with cooking, cleaning, getting to the doctor, and just getting out of the house. She helps them remember when to take their medications and how to follow their doctors' instructions. Burroughs said that helping these ladies is "very rewarding." Their children live in different cities, and Burroughs is often the only person nearby for them to talk to. When Burroughs goes out of town, she asks her relatives to step in and check on the ladies and see what they need. By cooking for the ladies, Burroughs has learned what they like. The 86-year-old, for example, loves bacon and croissants, cherry-cola, and caramel chocolate candy bars, and Burroughs said she has to hide the candy bars because otherwise the 86-year-old will eat them all at once. To take care of her own health, Burroughs goes to the gym three days a week and drinks fruit and vegetable smoothies for breakfast. Burroughs has to drive a considerable distance to see a specialist and said that she wishes there were more specialists available near her small town.

Warren Newton, the president and chief executive officer for the American Board of Family Medicine, observed that both Burroughs and Cruz embody the importance of social engagement and meaningful roles. Giving older adults the opportunity to be engaged in the community and to help other people is an essential part of healthy aging. Another workshop participant, Zohray Talib, the senior associate dean of academic affairs at the California University of Science and Medicine, added that in her work in Uganda and Kenya she has observed older people staying purposeful and engaged in their communities. There is a sense of community and support around older adults, and issues such as dementia are not pathologized but treated as normal behaviors. Talib described how a Kenyan woman spoke about her 90-year-old mother-in-law, who lives in a rural village and is busy with a sense of purpose and surrounded by family and grandchildren. However, Talib said, as people in these countries move to cities and become geographically dispersed, aging with a sense of purpose has become more difficult.

WORKING WITH OLDER ADULTS

Ricardo Custodio is a pediatrician and professor of health sciences based in Hawai'i. Hawai'i is a special place, Custodio said. It is geographically isolated, which has resulted in having an enormously biodiverse ecosystem and one of the most diverse, multiethnic, and multicultural populations in the world. There are a few Hawai'ian values that have been key to surviving and thriving, he said: aloha (love), malama (caring), and 'ohana (family). These values are expressed when you give the gift of flower lei to celebrate special occasions, including birthdays, weddings, graduations, and goodbyes. The elderly, called "kupuna," are celebrated in Hawai'i, he said. Custodio joked that you are officially elderly in Hawai'i when a cashier calls you "auntie" or "uncle" and automatically gives you the 10 percent discount. According to Custodio, the merging of Asian and Pacific Islander cultures means that "we malama our kupuna," or care for our elderly, because this is what 'ohana (family) does. He added that homes in Hawai'i are twice as likely to be multigenerational or more crowded than the national U.S. average, underscoring the concept of 'ohana, and "family means no one gets left behind or forgotten."

The values of aloha, malama, and 'ohana, Custodio said, are reflected in the fact that people living in Hawai'i have the longest life expectancy and are the happiest people in the United States (Arias et al., 2018; Mitchell et al., 2013). "We must be doing something differently and right to live longer and be happier," he said. The priority is to care for elders at home with the support of family and community, and it is a longstanding expectation that kupuna stay at home with their families. However, he added, not all people in Hawai'i enjoy this support. For example, when Custodio was a medical student in the emergency room, there was an elderly woman who would come in several times a week just to "talk story." She was the mother of a rich developer, but her son and grandchildren never came to visit; all the money in the world could not prevent her from being lonely, he said.

Custodio said he has spent his career trying to serve those who have been left behind, with a focus on providing health care to underserved children and families. His patients are primarily the poor, Pacific Islanders, and recently arrived non-English-speaking immigrants. For over 40 years Custodio has worked in community health centers that provide comprehensive services beyond primary care, regardless of patients' ability to pay. These services include homeless outreach, assistance with insurance eligibility, transportation, and translation as well as support from community health workers. More importantly, he said, these centers provide clerkships and training for health professions students to help them understand and experience what it is like to work in a community. The hope is to "brainwash" them into staying and committing to serve, he said. Over the last 12 years, Custodio has helped start a medical school, a nurse practitioner residency program, a clinical psychology fellowship, and a university division of natural and health sciences; all are focused on poor and underserved communities. These programs are part of his efforts focused on "growing our own, from our community, for our community." There are a huge number of health professions careers, and many are among the fastest growing occupations in the country. Training young people in these careers is a way to get underserved students into professions that can pay a living wage, he said.

Custodio noted that health professions training is often conducted in siloes and that upon entering practice, professionals are "thrown together" and expected to work like a team from day one. In sports, individuals learn individual skills but also spend dedicated time practicing and playing together as a team. "Why doesn't that happen in medicine?" he asked. He encouraged stakeholders to create a model of health professions education that consistently reminds students of the values of professionalism, teamwork, and service to the community. Clinical training centers should be created where students are given interprofessional health education directly in underserved communities. As an example of interprofessional training, Custodio spoke of how in the early 1990s a grant-funded project brought together medical, nursing, social work, and public health students for weekly sessions in a community health center. This experience instilled a sense of "community heart" in these students, he said.

Custodio also described a recent experience he had that showed him the power of love, caring, and family. He was hospitalized because he was urinating blood. He was in the hospital for several days receiving treatment, which gave him "a lot of time to think," he said. One reassuring insight he had concerned the strength of the community around him: the urologist was his former medical school classmate, the hospitalist was his former medical student, and the evening nurse was a former patient. The connections and support that he felt at his hospital gave him a sense that his community was rooting for him. The challenge, he said, is how to teach this to the next generation of health care providers. Where are the role models, and how can patients be guided to teach students about family and community? This is increasingly important to Custodio, he said, as he recently turned 65 and enrolled in Medicare.

Custodio discussed a number of trends relevant to the workshop. There is an increase in the number of older adults needing health care, while at the same time there is a decrease in the overall health care workforce due to retirement, death, and burnout. There is an increase in the amount of health care delivered at home rather than at hospitals and clinics. An interesting recent trend, he said, is that 85 to 90 percent of students going into health care are female, many of whom are immigrants, first-generation Americans, and minorities. This trend is in part due to the not-so-subtle advertising to caring, compassionate, and impressionable little girls; Custodio shared a picture of the wide variety of girl-oriented doctor toys and dolls that are available. This, he said, is how we make doctors. A more nurturing and caring workforce will change medicine for the better. The challenge for health professions education is to help young people define a purpose beyond the goal of acquiring material possessions and making money and toward social equity and justice, beyond the struggle for subsistence and toward serving others and building a sense of trust and hope for our kupuna.

During the pandemic, Custodio said that he felt this type of purpose and urgency in the younger generation. His clinic received a grant to train community contact tracers, with a focus on serving vulnerable populations; they had over 3,000 applications for 150 slots. Grades and degrees were important in choosing applicants, but the priority was to find candidates who had "community heart." Custodio described community heart as the "one kid who stays back and helps clean up" after everyone leaves a big family gathering. As health professions educators move forward in addressing the needs of an aging population, he said, there is a need to understand how individuals' development and their foundation of family and community affect their health and wellness. Providers need to actively encourage and seek out health professions candidates who have community heart, purpose, and desire to serve. The future that Custodio envisions is one in which older adults are healthy and are not alone because family and community are integrated into their care.

LEARNER RELUCTANCE

The global older adult population will double by 2050, said Cathy Maxwell of the Vanderbilt University School of Nursing. In the United States, the proportion of older adults will grow from 16 percent in 2021 to 22 percent in 2050 (ACL, 2021; WHO, 2022). In anticipation of this growth, the Institute of Medicine published a report in 2008 called *Retooling for an Aging America: Building a Healthcare Workforce* (IOM, 2008). Unfortunately, Maxwell said, the report did not have the desired impact. In fact, there has been a solid decline in geriatricians and nurse practitioners who work with older adults. Despite this report and other national initiatives—including the Eldercare Workforce Alliance, the Geriatric Workforce Enhancement Program, and the Nurses Improving Care for Health System Elders Program—the barriers to working with older adults have not been addressed. Maxwell reviewed a number of recent publications on aging adults and the health care workforce in order to lay a foundation for the rest of the workshop.

In April 2021, *Nature Aging* published a comment by John Rowe of Columbia University on the state of the U.S. eldercare workforce (Rowe,

2021). The piece included three major recommendations to improve the care of older adults, Maxwell said. First, Rowe urged a dramatic increase in the number of geriatric health care professionals, with a focus on public health professionals. Second, he advocated for population-focused and evidence-based policies and programs to support well-being. Third, Rowe addressed the need to implement recently formulated consensus recommendations regarding the care of community-dwelling older adults with serious illness. These recommendations included incorporating family members, applying technology, advancing cultural competency, and refining payment models.

One of the major barriers to expanding the workforce and improving the care of older adults, Maxwell said, is ageism among health care professionals as well as among older adults themselves. A study published in 2020 reported that not only does ageism exist, but it is well-established, socially accepted, and prevalent throughout the Western world (Chang et al., 2020). The study's authors advocated for educational interventions among clinicians to increase awareness of ageism, additional education and training to improve knowledge about aging, and research to explore factors related to the phenomenon of ageism among older adults. A 2019 special issue of the *Journal of the American Geriatric Society* addressed consensus-based recommendations for an adequate workforce, noting the need to use interprofessional teams; connect social, clinical, and home care services; build a culturally competent workforce; and train clinicians with appropriate communication skills (Spetz and Dudley, 2019). The special issue also emphasized the importance of the home care workforce, family caregiving, and palliative care.

A 2020 systematic review examined factors related to the preferences of students for working with older adults, Maxwell said (Hebditch et al., 2020). The review synthesized 62 papers and identified seven categories of factors that influence preferences, including student characteristics, experiences, courses, career, patient characteristics, and work characteristics. Maxwell described several key findings. First, during student training programs the preference for working with older adults actually decreases. The socialization process during these programs is seen as a deterrent and was referred to as a "hidden curriculum." The review noted there was a lack of educational interventions to address this hidden curriculum. A second key finding was that students had certain perceptions about the work, patients, and careers associated with working with older adults. Negative perceptions included a feeling that the work would be boring or emotionally challenging, the focus on quality of life rather than on curing patients, difficulties communicating with patients, and negative patient dispositions. Finally, the review identified the importance of exposure to healthy adults in order to reduce stereotypical prejudices and to promote working with older adults.

The National Hartford Center for Gerontological Nursing Excellence published core competencies for gerontological nursing educators in 2019 (NHCGNE, 2019). According to these findings, nursing educators should:

- Maintain knowledge and skills in the care of older adults
- Serve as advocates and positive role models for quality care for older adults
- Implement innovative teaching strategies for engaging learners to develop knowledge, attitudes, and skills for supporting healthy aging and the care of older adults
- Facilitate interprofessional learning opportunities related to healthy aging and care of older adults
- Facilitate the integration of concepts of healthy aging and care of older adults in academic and professional development programs
- Collaborate in the evaluation of learning about healthy aging and care of older adults in academic and professional development programs
- Demonstrate scholarship and leadership that advances gerontological nursing education and practice and that fosters others' professional development.

The "elephant in the room," Maxwell said, is the need for a paradigm shift in how students are taught to think about older adults and the ideas that shape our attitudes. Traditionally, she said, older adults are portrayed as frail, with fixed ideas of young versus old. There is a need to change learner attitudes about aging, Maxwell stated, before adding, "we don't have another decade to figure it out." Compounding the issue, she said, teachers are unlikely to engage in the type of collective change that is needed because of three factors: presentism, conservatism, and individualism. In a 1975 publication, Lortie described presentism as a focus on the short term, conservatism as a focus on small-scale achievements rather than broad change, and individualism as an idea that is reinforced by jobs with uncertain criteria for successful performance and reliance on their own indicators in isolation of a broader agenda (Nash and Ducharme, 1975).

Implementation science, to be discussed later, offers a path forward, Maxwell said. Implementation science is the study of the methods and strategies that facilitate the uptake of evidence-based practice and research into regular use by practitioners and policy makers (see Chapter 5 for more details). Maxwell said that a broader, holistic approach is needed in order to acknowledge the reality that aging is a process that begins early in life. The mechanisms of aging take place over decades, and most people have a long period with clinically healthy status. Once age-related pathologies appear, it is often too late to reverse the mechanisms of biological aging due to a lack of compensatory mechanisms and physiologic reserve. Maxwell compared the process to an iceberg, in which age-related pathologies are only the tip (Figure 1-1). There is a need, she said, to advance the understanding that aging is a continuum that begins around age 30, with a slow and incremental decline that is largely unnoticeable in younger and middle years. Later discussions at the workshop would focus more closely on how to shift attitudes and perceptions among learners in order to improve the capacity of the health care workforce to care for older adults.

INTRINSIC CAPACITY FRAMEWORK

The World Health Organization (WHO) articulated a vision for aging in 2016 (WHO, 2017). This vision, Maxwell said, represented a shift

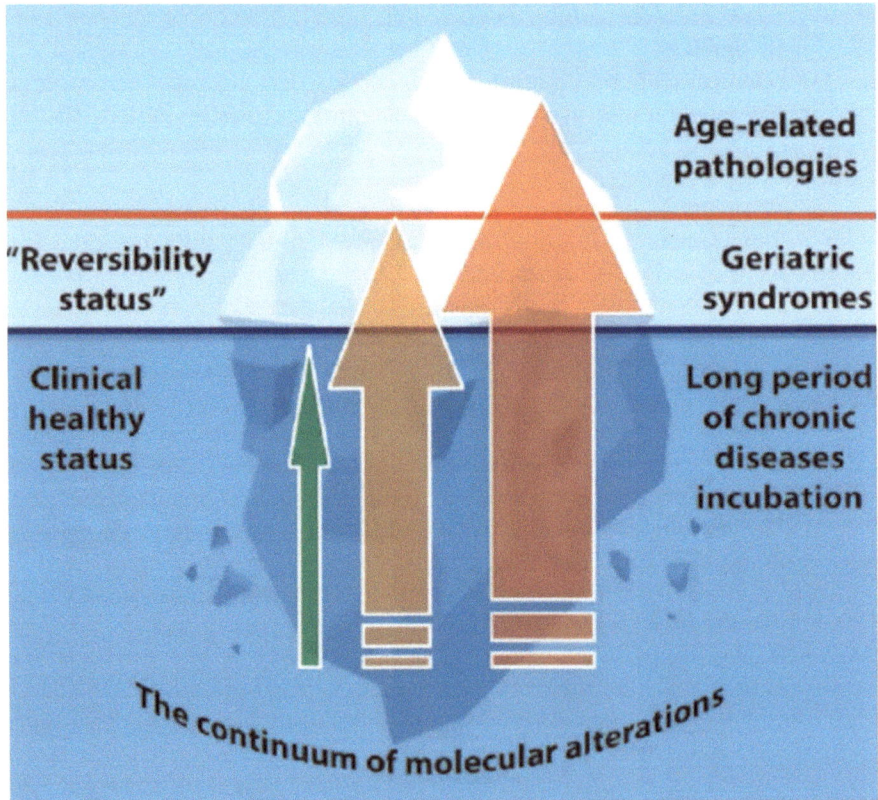

FIGURE 1-1 Iceberg model of aging.
SOURCES: Maxwell presentation, December 7, 2022; Franceschi et al. 2018.

away from thinking about health in older age as the presence or absence of disease and toward looking at functional ability. In addition, the vision endorsed the need for countries to cater more effectively to the needs of older people and to provide health services and care in a more integrated way. The intrinsic capacity (IC) framework comprises cognition, mobility, psychological, vitality, and sensory functions (Figure 1-2) (Zhou and Ma, 2022). Maxwell said that while this framework holds promise for mitigating functional decline, chronic conditions, and early mortality, it may not fully address other factors that contribute to harmonious aging. The harmonious aging approach, she explained, is designed to recognize the challenges and opportunities of old age, the tension between activity and disengagement, the integrity of the body and mind, and the interdependent nature of human beings. With this in mind, she, along with others involved in planning the workshop, suggested adding several factors to the intrinsic capacity framework: social, family, community, cultural, and spiritual. A roundtable of health professionals, students, and other stakeholders discussed the expanded IC framework and whether it is the right model to guide health care professionals in the care of older adults.

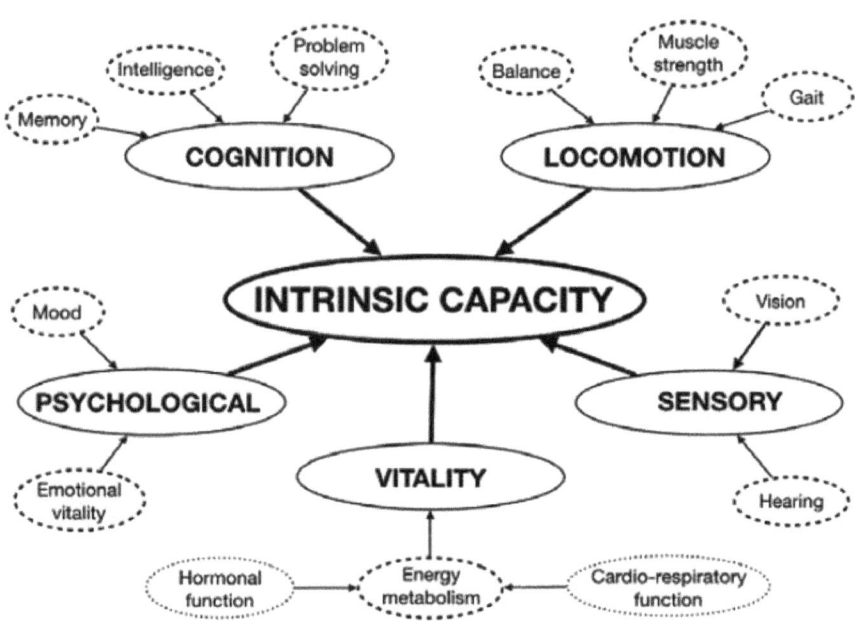

FIGURE 1-2 The World Health Organization's intrinsic capacity model for aging.
SOURCES: Presented by Maxwell, December 7, 2022; Cesari et al., 2018.

Integrative Health and Medicine Perspective

The IC model is an excellent one, said Liza Goldblatt, the director of national and global projects at the Academy of Integrative Health and Medicine, but it does focus mostly on the biological factors for aging. There are many other important areas that affect healthy aging, including social, cultural, community, economics, and family factors. Goldblatt said there are two movements that blend the IC model with the core values that Custodio discussed, such as family ties and cultural traditions. The first is the whole health movement, which began at the Department of Veterans Affairs and focuses on the whole person, including asking individuals what matters most to them and what their health priorities are. The second is the integrative health movement, which consists of conventional medicine providers working together with complementary medicine. Professionals in this movement include conventional medicine practitioners as well as acupuncturists, chiropractors, naturopathic physicians, Chinese medicine practitioners, and licensed massage therapists. Each of these disciplines addresses healthy aging and well-being as well as the treatment of diseases and conditions. These two movements, Goldblatt said, address the body, the mind, the emotions, the spirit, and the environment.

In 2014, a study found that over 30 percent of the U.S. population has access to integrated health care and that this percentage is even higher for seniors (Siddiqui et al., 2014). Since 2018 the Joint Commission has required hospitals to discuss non-pharmacological treatment of pain with patients. For example, patients who do not wish to be heavily sedated for pain management may be able to use acupuncture instead. Other options to improve the well-being of seniors include tai chi, chi gong, chiropractic care, mindfulness training, and nutritional strategies. However, conventional medical systems are still largely unaware of these disciplines, their philosophies, and their scopes of practice. This is a significant gap in health professions education and practice in the United States. The current health care system, Goldblatt said, is not set up for optimal health and well-being. It is designed more for the treatment of diseases, which, while being an important part of health care, is limited. Since so many diseases are preventable, she asked, is it not time to also put the country's economic resources towards supporting the creation of good health? Health professionals are dedicated and motivated, but they simply cannot address the needs of patients in 15-minute visits in a for-profit medical system. As Cruz observed in the first session of the workshop, health professionals are not given the time they need with patients. "We need to change our health care system" if there will be any impact on the health and well-being of the aging population, Goldblatt said.

Nutrition Perspective

Food and nutrition touch all of the five original domains of the IC framework as well as the factors that the planning committee suggested adding, said Kathy Kolasa, a professor emerita at East Carolina University's Brody School of Medicine. While not everyone can share the beautiful flowers of Hawai'i, she said, people around the globe share food with their families and friends as a way of expressing love and caring. Food is an important component of the IC framework, although it is rarely mentioned in the literature. Kolasa gave three reasons why nutrition should be considered in all domains of the IC framework. First, frailty and malnutrition are established risk factors for loss of function (Cesari et al., 2018). Roughly 22 percent of older adults in the hospital and approximately 30 percent of those in long-term care are malnourished, which has an impact on their recovery and function. Second, activities of daily living (ADLs) are discussed in the IC literature, but there is a need for more emphasis on the instrumental ADLs, such as accessing and preparing food (Zhou and Ma, 2022). Health professionals can screen for food insecurity in clinical settings and can help connect people to the resources they need. Dietitians can counsel patients on how to get a good-quality diet, which is important for retaining function. Third, Kolasa said, many chronic disease conditions have a nutrition component, and about 50 percent of older Americans are obese (Jimenez et al., 2022). The standard advice given to young people for weight loss may not be effective for older adults and could even lead to loss of function. Registered dietitian nutritionists can conduct nutritional assessments and promote the adoption of preventive strategies for aging that address frailty, disability, and other issues that matter most to older adults. Kolasa said that weight loss is sometimes discouraged for older adults because of fears of making function worse, but the things that matter most to older adults often require weight loss. For example, an individual may want to run around with his or her grandchildren or get up off the floor independently. Weight loss can be done safely and appropriately and should not be discouraged for this population, Kolasa said. She added that a focus on function for older adults can be an opportunity to bring together professionals from different specialties; for example, occupational therapy students and dietetic students could work together to help patients use adaptive tools to cook and eat healthy meals.

Medical Perspective

The model of care in both the United States and around the world is disease-centered, said Senthil Rajasekaran, the associate dean and chief academic officer at Khalifa University College of Medicine and Health

Sciences. However, for the geriatric population in particular, the ideal model of care is function-centered, with an emphasis on issues that matter to the individual. Functional ability is determined primarily by the intrinsic capacity—that is, the composite of all of the physical and mental capacities of the individual—along with the environment. The five domains of the IC framework are pivotal for capturing an individual's intrinsic capacity, he said. Unfortunately, he added, the health professions education system does not adequately address these topics or focus on function-based care. The growth in the population of older adults is not being matched by a growth in relevant areas of health education. It is critical, he said, that the health professions education system "takes a huge stride" in including a significant amount of educational material that will help learners be prepared to take care of the elderly population when they enter clinical practice. There are a variety of methods to introduce this content, he said, including simulations, gamification, and opportunities for students to "roll up their sleeves" and work in the community with older adults. The current generation is motivated to make an impact in their community, Rajasekaran said, so there need to be opportunities for them to do so.

Learner Perspective

A doctoral student in nursing practice within adult geriatrics at Vanderbilt University, Brooke Hazen commented that there is not much emphasis on the duty within the health care system to serve others. Specifically, she said, patients are seen as separate from providers, and providers do not see taking care of patients as a way of making their own lives better. Hazen said that while there have been many efforts to improve the health care system—for example, to make it more cost-effective or more evidence-based—there is a need for a mindset shift toward a value-based system. Health professionals need to be given the time and training to act as patient advocates, and they need to think of themselves as advocates. The "whole country" needs to push back on our current system, she said, and demand a change. As a student, Hazen said, she has had the opportunity to meet with patients for long periods of time, to listen to their issues, and to identify multiple ways that their health and care could be improved. No one else in the system is catching these things, she said, because they simply do not have the time to see the big picture. There is a need for a major shift within health professions education and practice in order to provide patient-centered care that addresses the whole person.

Hazen also spoke of the importance of interprofessional training and practice. Part of her nurse practitioner training included a 2-year clinical program in which nursing students worked on teams that included medical, pharmacy, social work, divinity, and counseling students. The teams worked in clinics and also visited older adults in their homes. Hazen emphasized the value of this interprofessional training, saying it was the highlight moment for her in terms of how she provides care and how she sees health care.

Community Perspective

Zohray Talib of the California University of Science and Medicine agreed with other speakers about the need for a cultural shift within the health care system. The question, she said, is what will this mean for health professions educators and what actions need to be taken? Talib described three levels at which changes need to be made. First, at the macro level there is a need for new policies and an evolution of accreditation and regulatory requirements. These changes cannot wait, she said, because the demographic shift is already happening. At the institutional level, institutions need to be responsive to the needs of an aging population and should incorporate the perspective of older individuals in leadership and governance. Furthermore, many educators themselves are older adults, so institutions need to be thinking about issues such as retirement and burnout. At the learner level, students need to move into the community and learn from older adults directly. Talib said that the discussions at the workshop have made her feel inspired, but she also feels a sense of urgency to act. There is a need to start visualizing what success looks like and what steps can be taken to get there, she concluded.

Psychology Perspective

Health professions education often focuses on disease, said Catherine Grus, the chief education officer at the American Psychological Association, but there is a need to shift the perspective toward health promotion. Training health professionals to think about how to promote health and well-being in older adults can make a big impact, she said. For example, several speakers mentioned the issue of loneliness in older adults. Loneliness can progress to depression, and there are high rates of suicide in older adults (Crestani et al., 2019). Taking a health promotion perspective can lead one to intervene early and mitigate against the progression of the depression. However, the current health care workforce does not have the capacity to take this approach, she said, and educators are "not going to get there overnight." Another critical piece of caring for older adults, Grus added, is using an interdisciplinary approach and working closely with professionals across the spectrum. For example, if an individual presents with symptoms of depression, it is imperative to work with other professionals to discern whether the depression is related to a medical condition or perhaps is an early stage of cognitive decline. In psychology in particular, she said, there is a lack of emphasis on health promotion and the role of communities in promoting and supporting well-being.

Social Work Perspective

The IC framework fits nicely with the social work perspective, said Nancy Kusmaul of the University of Maryland School of Social Work. For generations, social work has taught the person and environment model, which looks at the interaction between the environment and the individual's strengths and challenges, including physical, mental, cognitive, emotional, and spiritual issues. The problem, however, is getting social work students interested in working with older adults. Offering separate classes on older adults is not particularly effective, she said, because the only students who enroll are those who are already interested in working with this population. Kusmaul added that while students may say they want to work with families and children, they do not generally think about the fact that older adults are part of families. Connecting students with older adults through the classroom or practical experiences, she said, is one approach to get students interested. She commented on hearing from multiple practitioners that "accidental experience" with older adults is what got them interested in the field. Kusmaul urged health professions educators to think of ways to expose students to older adults in order to spark interest and improve care for this population.

2

Exploring What Matters Most in Working with Older Adults

Key Messages Made by Presenters

- The first step of the process [in the course] is for students to get to know older adults and to understand what matters to them. (Lynch)
- The four Ms in the program stand for what matters, medication, mentation (mental activity and stimulation), and mobility. Students should be taught early about the four Ms and how they will be expected to deliver 4Ms care both during and after their education. (Pohnert, Dolansky)

Multiple individual speakers at the workshop emphasized the importance of focusing on what matters most to older adults. In the two sessions described in this chapter, presenters discussed programs that seek to do so. The first presentation described a course in which students work closely with older adults in the community to address some of their challenges. The second presentation described the 4Ms approach for age-friendly health systems and explains how it was implemented at CVS MinuteClinics.

ENGINEERING FOR HUMANITY

People are at the center of everything, said Caitrin Lynch, the dean of faculty and a professor of anthropology at Olin College of Engineering. When innovating or trying to make change, it is critical to "hold on to what really matters to people" and create things that are relevant and useful. This people-first principle is the heart of a class that Lynch teaches called Engineering for Humanity. The course is based on the innovator's compass (Figure 2-1), which was created by Lynch's colleague Ela Ben-Ur. The course is interdisciplinary, Lynch said, and students receive half their credits in anthropology and half in engineering. Students come from three different colleges—Olin College of Engineering, Wellesley College, and Babson College—and are placed in teams with an older adult community partner. These partnerships are facilitated through a longstanding relationship with the Council on Aging, she said.

The course was first developed with a grant from a local health care foundation with the aim of creating an opportunity for engineering students to work with older people to design tools that would help people stay in

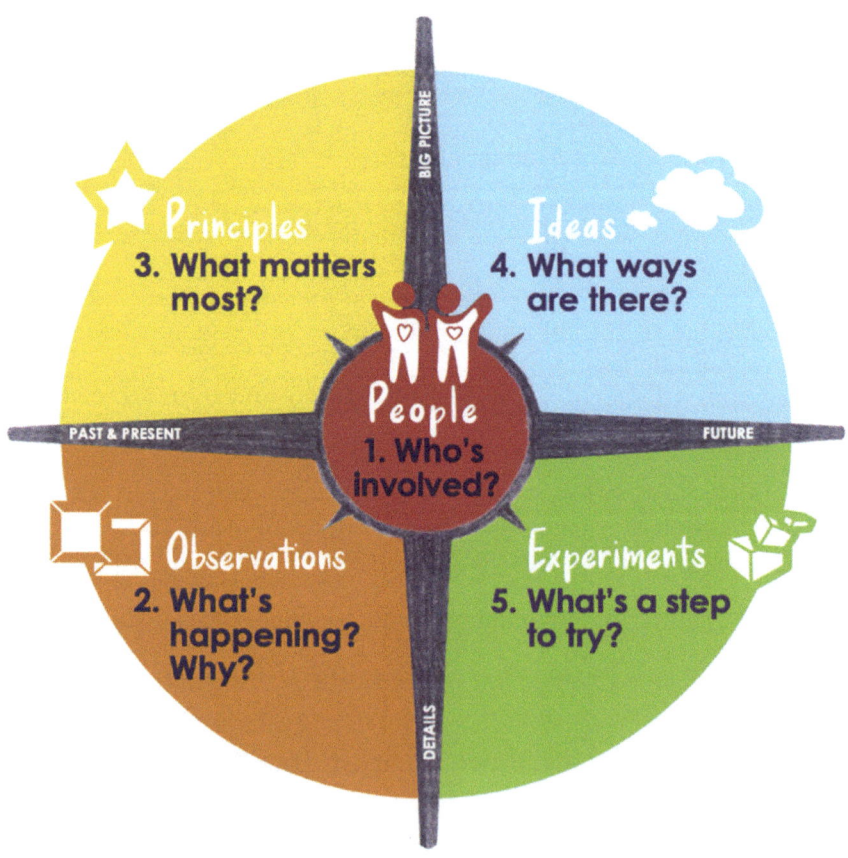

FIGURE 2-1 Innovator's compass.
SOURCES: Lynch presentation, December 8, 2022; Ben-Ur, 2020.

their homes and live independently. The first step of the process, Lynch said, is for students to get to know the older adults and to understand what matters to them. Using the iterative innovator's compass, the students immerse themselves in the lives of their senior partners and come up with ideas to help people achieve their goals. For example, students may go to movies with their partners, go shopping, or play chair volleyball in a senior center. Lynch offered the example of one student team that went grocery shopping with an older adult named Terry who uses a wheelchair and has hearing loss. In the second step of the compass, the students observed that Terry had issues with reaching and carrying groceries at the store as well as challenges in her home. In the third step, the students identified the principles that were important to Terry, namely, independence, social engagement, and positivity. The students brainstormed multiple potential ideas, including a tool to help Terry reach groceries, a way for her to use her oven, and multi-modal alarms in her home. Many plans and prototypes were produced, and the students ultimately focused on helping Terry get her groceries from the store. One approach that could have been taken, Lynch said, would be to stack four bags of groceries on the back of the wheelchair to maximize convenience and efficiency. However, going to the store was an important activity for Terry, given her desire for social engagement. Thus, instead of maximizing efficiency, the students maximized social engagement by producing a system that would help Terry carry two bags of groceries on the back of her chair. Students used a "prototype, pilot, produce" iterative process to develop the final product. The product included communication symbols and served as a point of conversation at the store, which meant that Terry was able to do what mattered most to her and spend her time engaging with those around her.

Lynch shared several other examples of designs that students created during the course, including a tool to help a man with diabetic neuropathy massage his own feet instead of waking his wife to massage them, a device that magnified photos for a woman with macular degeneration who liked to tell stories about her photos, and a cutting board with physical guides for a woman with vision problems who loved to cook. Lynch emphasized that although the class helps students develop their engineering skills, the focus is on understanding people and what matters to them. "Engineering skills include people skills," she said, just as health professionals need training in listening to people and understanding their experiences. Furthermore, the type of creativity used in the program is not confined to engineers or designers. People in any profession can use a system like the innovator's compass to observe and figure out what really matters to people and how to address those needs.

Lynch was joined by two students from the course along with their community partner, Peggy, to share their story. The project began during the COVID-19 pandemic, said one of the students, Ian Eykamp, which meant that initial meetings were held over Zoom. During these sessions, the team learned about Peggy, her family, and her routine. Eykamp emphasized that it was important to learn about all aspects of Peggy because without this knowledge, it would have been difficult to know what would be useful. One challenge that Peggy told the students about was difficulty carrying laundry down the stairs. Over Zoom, she described the problem and shared pictures and video of her staircase and railing. The students and Peggy brainstormed ideas, which included a laundry chute, a "mini ski lift," a tristar wheel stair climbing basket, a pulley system, and a sled attached to the railings. Eykamp said that Peggy "was full of great suggestions and solutions" and that it was critical to get her firsthand perspective as the person who actually experienced the challenge and needed a solution. The students performed experiments, tried out concepts in sketch models, and developed prototypes. As COVID vaccines became available, the team was able to visit Peggy in her home and have her try out some of the potential solutions. The final product was a device that holds a laundry basket and slides down the railing. Zoie Leo, another student member of the team, added that a plastic stopper at the bottom of the railing was central to the design and said that it was only possible to add this component because they were working in the specific space that they were designing for.

Peggy Wihtol, the team's community partner, told workshop participants about her experience in the Engineering for Humanity class. Wihtol retired at 62 and enjoyed an active retirement, volunteering at a food pantry and a nursing home, working part-time, and traveling with her husband. In 2014 her husband began showing signs of Alzheimer's, and she soon became his full-time caregiver. He entered a nursing home in late 2019 and died of COVID-19 in early 2020. The pandemic left Wihtol in isolation at home, with no caregiving responsibilities or volunteer responsibilities. Friends called and checked on her, but she mostly stayed home due to COVID. She joked that her dog did not learn to speak English, no matter how much she talked to her. By January 2021, Wihtol said, she was "desperate" for something to do, and she learned about the opportunity to participate in the class. She was very happy to have people to talk to and to learn from, she said, although the class was "unlike any college class" she had ever taken. One of the first things that happened was that she received a brown box at the door full of "strange stuff" like paper towel rolls, pipe cleaners, clay, fabric, and Post-it Notes. The first Zoom class felt like "speed dating," with everyone trying to get to know each other. Wihtol said she appreciated the emphasis on finding ways to stay in her home, because after 50 years in the same house, moving out would be harder than staying.

Wihtol and the students got to know each other over Zoom; she was interested in the people on her team, and she found that they had things in common. The students and Wihtol bonded over their interests in travel, dogs, the outdoors, cooking, education, and business, and some of the students had relatives with Alzheimer's. Wihtol's main concern that she wanted addressed was her safety, particularly on the stairs. The team batted around many ideas, and she nixed some of them based on concerns about safety or due to the layout of her home. Wihtol said that she came up with the idea of the stair rail rider and felt "very responsible" for the ultimate design. The process required a lot of trust, she said, particularly because everyone was working remotely due to COVID. Each student found his or her own niche of responsibility and own way to communicate with Wihtol. She said that she tried to be "gentle" when she communicated with the students, particularly when she was shooting down one of their ideas. The students taught Wihtol how to use new technologies, such as Google Slides, and she taught herself new things as well. She is still in touch with some of the students and has visited their colleges. Wihtol read the summary she wrote at the end of the project:

> *My thanks to Olin, the Engineering for Humanity faculty, the students on Team Peg. I had been in a rough place with COVID and the loss of my husband, and needed something new and interesting to invest in and concentrate on. This was it. The pleasure of working with young, ambitious, caring students, a faculty and facility which so strongly believes in hands-on learning and fostering community relationships, and all of the Engineering for Humanity program has renewed my soul and re-engaged my brain.*

AGE-FRIENDLY HEALTH SYSTEMS AND THE 4MS FRAMEWORK

Mary Dolansky, a professor in the School of Nursing at Case Western Reserve University, and Ann Pohnert, the lead director of clinical quality at CVS MinuteClinic, told workshop participants about their experience implementing the 4Ms age-friendly health systems framework in CVS MinuteClinics. Age-Friendly Health Systems is an initiative aimed at ensuring that older adults receive evidence-based care in every setting, from hospitals to primary care to convenient care settings, Pohnert said. There are many evidence-based geriatric care models that have been proven effective, she continued, but only a small proportion of these are reaching those who could benefit. This is due, she said, to the fact that it can be difficult to disseminate and scale models and to reproduce performance in settings with fewer resources, and models may not translate across care settings. The 4Ms is an evidence-based framework for age-friendly care that was developed by geriatric experts. These experts identified four essential sets of evidence-based practices that cause no harm, can be used by anyone, and are consistent with what matters most to older adults and their families. The aim of the 4Ms movement was to reach older adults in 2,600 hospitals, practices, clinics, and nursing homes by June 30, 2023; Pohnert said the goal had already been exceeded as of December 2022. One partner in the initiative is CVS MinuteClinics, which are care clinics located in CVS stores. There are about 1,100 clinics in 36 states; these clinics see about 6 million patients per year, including 1 million older adults. Clinics are staffed by nurse practitioners and physician assistants and are accredited by the Joint Commission. The care at MinuteClinics is less expensive than traditional care, Pohnert said, in part because there are fewer overhead costs. These clinics serve as a safety net for the community, and there is a high rate of patient satisfaction.

The four Ms in the 4Ms program refer to what matters, medication, mentation, and mobility (Figure 2-2). Each setting that implements the 4Ms program may define them slightly differently, depending on the patient population and their needs, Pohnert said. She described each of the four Ms in turn. The first M is "what matters." This means that providers need to know and understand each individual's specific health outcome goals and care preferences and to align care with these needs. In the CVS MinuteClinic context, this entails having a discussion about what matters in every visit (except for vaccinations and express visits for COVID), asking patients what matters, documenting what they say, and acting upon it. The second M is "medication." If medications are necessary for a patient, the 4Ms framework encourages the use of age-friendly medications that do not interfere with the other Ms (what matters, mentation, and mobility). At the MinuteClinic, Pohnert said, this means checking medications against the American Geriatric Society Beers list of medications that may not be appropriate for older adults and discussing with the patient ways to make medication use safer, e.g., using pillboxes, education, and deprescribing. The third M is "mentation," which has two parts. The first is depression, which MinuteClinics screen for using the PhQ-2 and PhQ-9. Based on the results of the screening, the provider may provide a brochure, educate the patient, or refer the patient to an appropriate outside provider. The second part of mentation is dementia; MinuteClinics screen for dementia using the Mini-Cog© and educate or refer patients to other providers or resources. Finally, the fourth M is "mobility." The aim of this piece is to ensure that each older adult moves safely every day to maintain function and to do what matters most. MinuteClinics use a Modified Timed Get Up and Go test to assess mobility, and they may provide patients with a brochure, further education, or a referral. All screening results and actions taken are documented in the electronic health record, Pohnert said.

Although each of the four Ms is important in and of itself, Pohnert said, they are meant to be assessed as a set. Over the last 3 years at CVS

EXPLORING WHAT MATTERS MOST IN WORKING WITH OLDER   23

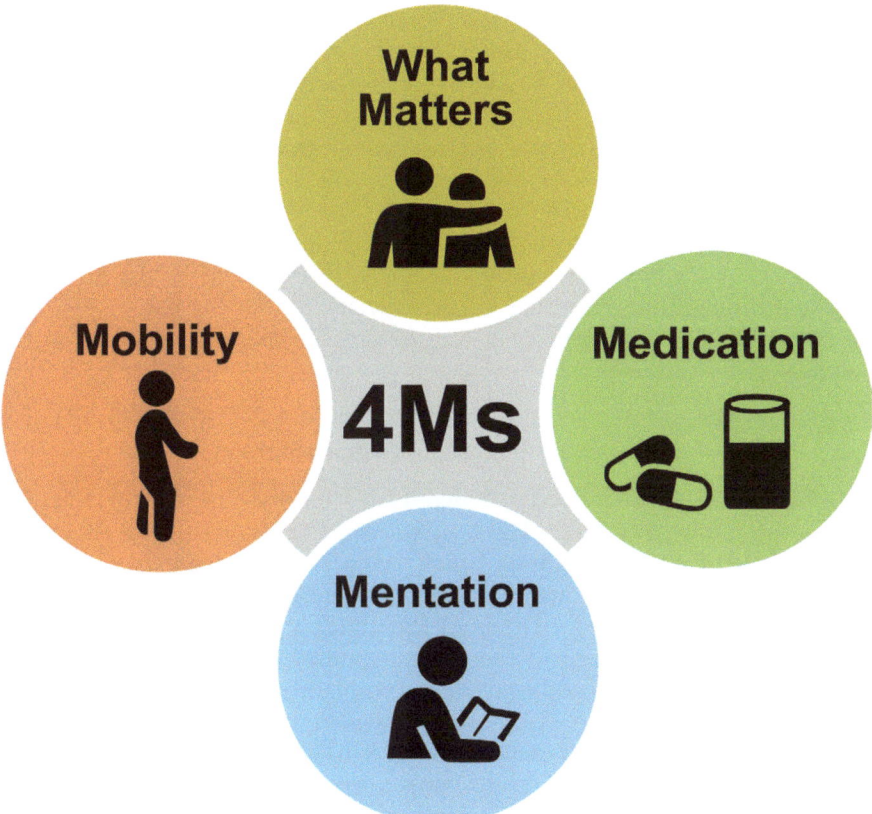

FIGURE 2-2 The four Ms of age-friendly health systems.
SOURCE: Pohnert presentation, December 8, 2022; Institute for Healthcare Improvement, 2023, *Age-friendly health systems*. https://www.ihi.org/Engage/Initiatives/Age-Friendly-Health-Systems/Pages/default.aspx (accessed April 22, 2023). Used with permission.

MinuteClinics, there have been over 40,000 visits in which all four Ms were used, and over 370,000 visits in which at least one M was used. Throughout this time period, the proportion of visits with the use of all four Ms has increased significantly, and progress has also been seen in increased visit times for older adults. Pohnert shared a real-life example of how the process works. A 75-year-old female came into the clinic to be evaluated and treated for a sinus infection. The nurse practitioner who treated her looked at her medical history and talked to her about what mattered to her—in this case, family togetherness and health. She moved around well, although she expressed concerns about living alone and falling. The nurse practitioner discussed eliminating clutter and other safety issues around the home. Two of her medications were flagged as potential concerns, and she reported that she had already spoken with her primary provider about them; he indicated she could not reduce or eliminate either medication. On a memory assessment, the patient had difficulty recalling words and reported that she was concerned about her short-term memory. The nurse practitioner added a neurology referral to the record and urged the patient to talk to her primary provider as well as her family. The patient, Pohnert said, was very happy with her care and very appreciative for the extra time and attention. While the visit was for a specific illness, the patient was able to receive support and care for a number of issues because of the tools and support given to the clinician.

Implementation and Educational Strategies

After Pohnert described the details of the 4Ms program, Dolansky discussed implementation of the program. The approach taken to implement the 4Ms into MinuteClinics has bearing on how to implement geriatrics concepts into health professions education and residency, she said. Dolansky described a number of methods and frameworks that were used to expand the reach of the 4Ms, including the learning health care organization, quality improvement, and implementation science. Learning health care organizations are those that are willing to learn and improve; educational organizations must also be willing to learn and improve in order to implement new ideas and approaches. The quality improvement efforts, Dolansky said, were led by the director of clinical quality, who established a quality improvement infrastructure. In clinical practice, she said, a lot of change can be facilitated by the data generated by the electronic health record; educational organizations also need infrastructure in order to use quality improvement approaches. The plan–do–study–act (PDSA) philosophy can be used in small test cycles to reflect on and make changes, she said. The implementation science approaches that were used, Dolansky said, included the Consolidated Framework for Implementation Science (CFIR), the RE-AIM evaluation framework, and the Expert Recommendations for Implementing Change (ERIC). Dolansky encouraged education stakeholders to look to implementation science in order to make changes in their own systems. Dolansky also shared the logic model used for implementing the 4Ms into the CVS MinuteClinics (Figure 2-3); she noted that the tenets of the RE-AIM model (reach, effectiveness, adoption, implementation, and maintenance) guided the development of the logic model.

There are three major components of implementation strategies that are critical for making change, Dolansky said: infrastructure, practice-based

Age-Friendly Health Systems Convenient Care Continuum Logic Model

Objective: to extend the reach and impact of Age-Friendly Health Systems principles within convenient care settings. **Opportunity:** to develop a plan to implement the Age-Friendly Health Systems initiative within the CVS MinuteClinic health system. *denotes an output, process, or outcome measure designated by the IHI Guidelines

INPUTS	ACTIVITIES →	OUTPUTS →	OUTCOMES
What we invest (resources)	What we do:	Direct products of program activities	Changes in behavior, knowledge, attitudes, conditions:
FTE/staff	Maintenance of virtual clinic and educational platform Implementation Strategies	1. Virtual clinic (NP time spent in virtual clinic, NP competency) 2. Educational platform (# of sessions attended; # of NPs trained) 3. Practice-based implementation strategies	**Care Delivery** • NP 4Ms actions are conducted for all eligible patients (compliance rate) • Delivery of 4Ms care within standard times allotments
Faculty experts			
Partners: CVS, IHI, John Hartford Foundation	Age-Friendly "4Ms" EPIC System Integration	7. # of 4Ms assessments and prevalence rates (including what matters, medications, dementia, depression, mobility documentation)* 8. # of provider 4Ms related act-ons – referrals, further testing, educational materials, deprescribing, integration of what matters 9. # of NPs that deliver all 4Ms assessments and # of act-ons 10. Counts and rates (%) of people receiving all 4Ms (volume) < 65, 65-74, 75-84, 85+ years and according to race/ethnicity* 11. Practice based tool kits – # of brochures given to patients 12. Revisions to the EPIC system workflow and screens	**Satisfaction** • Maintained patient satisfaction with using CVS • Increased # of older adults >65 using MC • Increased # of people coming back for services **Health** • Decrease in prescribed, high-risk medications (i.e., AGS and Beers)
Technology			
Collaborating institutions: Rush University			
Consultants			
Front-line support (DNP Fellows, informants)	Patient and NP Surveys	13. collaboRATE – participant survey of care concordance with what matters* 14. Impact on Care Team – two qualitative questions completed by NPs*	**Transitions of care (hubs sites)** • Decreased Emergency Department (ED) visits*
Champions	Develop and evaluate two booster trainings	15. Create PDSA and Virtual Clinic booster training materials 16. Feasibility survey on booster trainings 17. Self-efficacy and/or reflective practice survey on booster trainings 18. Qualitative feedback on booster training experience	

Updated: 2/22/2022

FIGURE 2-3 Logic model for implementation of age-friendly health systems principles within convenient care settings.
SOURCE: Dolansky presentation, December 8, 2022.

tools, and professional development. At MinuteClinics, the infrastructure that supports implementation of the 4Ms includes data analytics, performance evaluations, virtual huddles, advisories and newsletters, an electronic message board, and the clinical dashboard. These mechanisms for support and feedback are essential for improvement.

A practice-based tool to support implementation of the 4Ms is the EPIC health record system, which includes a 4M Age-Friendly Evaluation tab and a pocket card that can be given to patients to help them understand age-friendly care. Another useful tool for the 4Ms is a patient brochure that reviews the purpose and history of age-friendly health systems, introduces the 4Ms, and leaves space for the practitioner to document action steps for each M. A process map was developed to help practitioners automatically integrate the 4Ms into their usual primary care visit (Figure 2-4). These types of tools, Dolansky said, would also be helpful for learners in the delivery of geriatrics care in different practice settings.

Professional development was also a critical piece of implementing 4Ms into MinuteClinics, Dolansky said. A variety of platforms and activities were used to reach and educate practitioners, including monthly grant rounds, optional video vignettes, education exchange on "hot topics," acknowledging age-friendly health system champions, clinical education resources, and a weekly newsletter. One challenge that some of the early career nurse practitioners have, Dolansky said, is a lack of confidence in patient communication. In order to address this, a Confident Conversations tool was created which helps guide providers through the conversations they need to have about the 4Ms. In addition, providers are given a decision tree to help guide their actions after assessment (Figure 2-5), and there is a "virtual clinic" for practitioners to practice and assess their competency in the 4Ms. Virtual clinical practice is an excellent opportunity to expose students to geriatric care, she said.

Interprofessional Implications

The 4Ms is a national movement, and it is important that students, residents, and practitioners all be on board, Dolansky said. In all disciplines, students should be taught early about the 4Ms and how they will be expected to deliver 4Ms care both during and after their education. The Institute for Healthcare Improvement (IHI) has created a module for all health care professionals to learn age-friendly care; this is an excellent resource to prime students on geriatric care (IHI, 2020). At Case Western Reserve University, students from multiple health professions programs can participate in a certificate program for age-friendly learning; the program includes the IHI module and small group discussions about interprofessional collaboration on the 4Ms and uses a virtual clinic. Students are

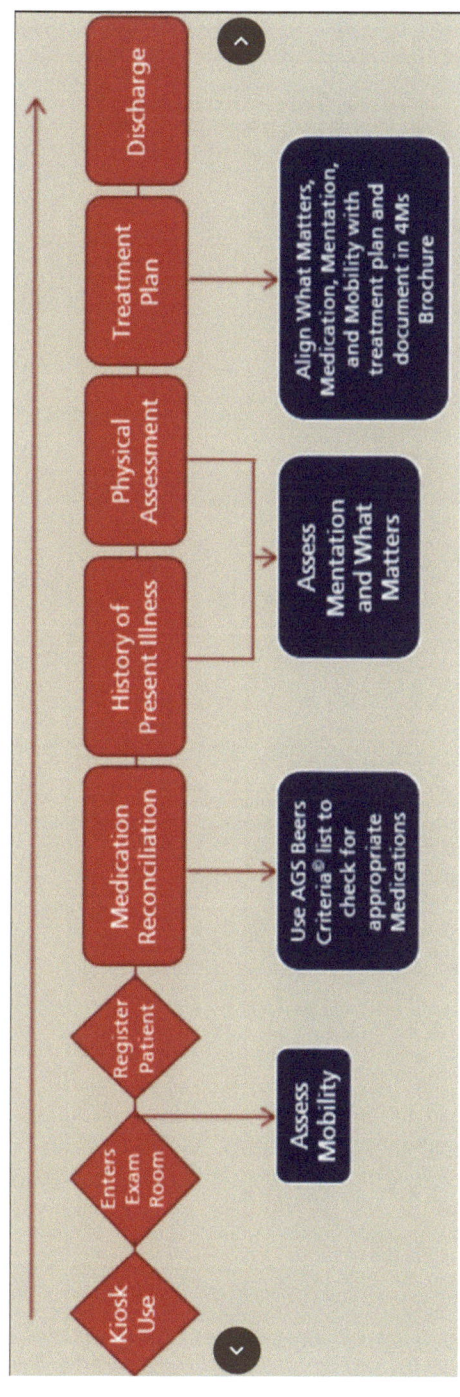

FIGURE 2-4 Process map for implementation of 4Ms in primary care visit.
SOURCE: Dolansky presentation, December 8, 2022.

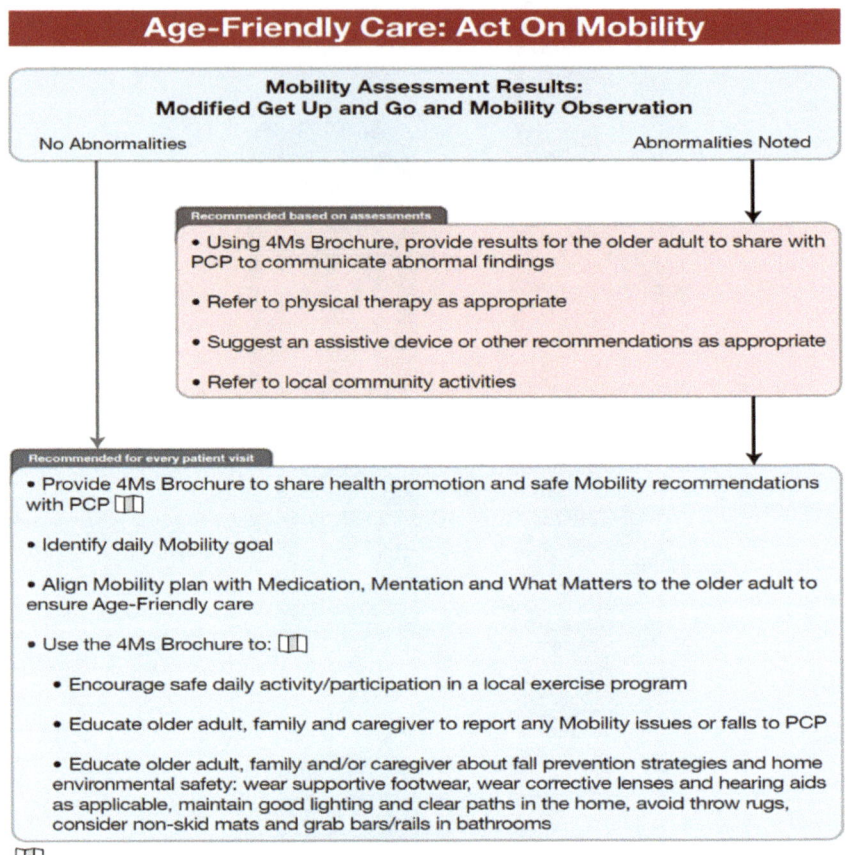

FIGURE 2-5 Act-on decision tree for mobility.
SOURCE: Dolansky presentation, December 8, 2022.

generally technologically savvy, Dolansky noted, and the virtual environment offers an opportunity to educate and train students on experiences they may not get in their practice settings. Embracing these types of educational opportunities, she said, will allow students to have a robust experience along the continuum of aging and to embrace the joy of the delivery of care for older adults.

3

Supply and Demand: Is the Workforce Prepared to Meet the Needs of Older Adults?

Key Messages Made by Presenters

- These numbers mean that the population will be more advanced in age and more racially diverse, with an older workforce, while Alzheimer's is projected to increase by 116 percent. (George)
- Ageism itself may deter students from wanting to work in geriatrics or gerontology. Furthermore, implicit or explicit bias among faculty in health professions education programs can push students in other directions. (Hartley)
- The trainees left the clinic each day challenged by the complexity of the care and also with a high degree of satisfaction because they felt they were really helping the older adults. (Bradley, Mazzurco, Lawrence)
- Incentives—particularly financial incentives—are important to the efforts to increase the workforce and improve senior care. However, they are often seen as a panacea. (Moone)

Greg Hartley, an associate professor of clinical physical therapy and medical education at the University of Miami, moderated this session of the workshop, which focused on whether the supply (i.e., the health care workforce) is or will be adequate to meet the demand (i.e., the need for care of older adults). This session was divided into three parts, Hartley explained, beginning with a presentation detailing how the population of the United States is changing, what the health care needs of U.S. citizens will be, and who will be needed to provide care and in what settings. The second part emphasized ageism within push and pull factors that draw people toward or away from working with older adults. Finally, Hartley said, part three of the session would gather input from individuals representing a variety of professional backgrounds to reflect and build upon what they heard in the previous presentations.

HEALTH CARE NEEDS AND CAREGIVER SUPPLY

Over the next roughly 40 years, said Rebecca George, an M.D. candidate at the University of California Davis, the U.S. population is expected to grow by 22 percent to 404 million (Vespa et al., 2020). There will be a 92 percent increase in the population of adults who are 65 and older and a nearly 618 percent increase in the number of centenarians (Vespa et al., 2020). The population will be increasingly diverse, with the majority of the population being people from ethnic and racial minorities. In addition to these general population demographic changes, the makeup of the labor force is also changing, George said. The proportion of younger workers will decrease, while the proportion of older workers will increase. Taken together, she said, these numbers mean that the population will be more advanced in age and more racially diverse, with an older workforce. This presents an opportunity, she added, for more cultural humility[1] and understanding of the various intersections of identity of the patients when engaging with them. As a result of the aging population, the prevalence of conditions such as diabetes, stroke, heart failure, and hypertension will increase by around 33 percent, while Alzheimer's is projected to increase by 126 percent (Alzheimer's Association, 2023; Roth, 2022). Currently, the population of older adults who are providing formal and informal health care are overwhelmingly female (61 percent), mostly over 75 years old (74 percent), and around a quarter live alone (AARP, 2020). Care recipients primarily need care for long-term physical conditions, memory, short-term physical ailments, and mental health.

Those who care for older adults can be lay people or health care professionals. A 2020 study by AARP and the National Alliance for Caregiving found that almost 19 percent of adults are lay caregivers, George said, and this number is likely to increase as the population ages. Further noted in the report is that lay caregivers are primarily female and over 50 years old; 89 percent of caregivers are a relative of those they care for. About a quarter of caregivers are caring for multiple adults, and 14 percent have been caregiving for more than 10 years. COVID-19, with its impacts on

---

[1] Cultural humility is a term used to describe personal relationships that honor another person's beliefs, customs, and values; and requires continuous self-exploration and self-critique while learning from others (Stubbe, 2020).

mental and physical health, has changed the care landscape in ways that are still being accounted for, she added.

The health care workforce is projected to grow by 13 percent over the next 10 years, adding roughly 2 million jobs (BLS, 2022). This growth will vary greatly by discipline, George said. Disciplines that are projected to grow by at least 25 percent include nurse practitioners, physician assistants, home health aides, and occupational therapy assistants and aides. At the other end, the number of dentists, registered nurses, psychologists, and physicians is expected to grow by 6 percent or less. George emphasized that these data reflect the growth in the field and do not speak to whether this growth is adequate to meet the demand for care. The location of health care delivery is shifting as well, she said, with direct care worker projected job openings in home care expected to increase by 37 percent between 2020 and 2023 and by 22 percent in residential care homes during the same period (PHI, 2023).

The health care professions' educational system is where these future professionals will be trained. At present, George said, the United States has almost 20,000 health care training programs at nearly 9,000 sites (not specific to geriatrics). More than 50 percent of these programs are graduate-level training programs, of which more than half are physician residencies. This number is at odds with the fact that physicians are one of the slowest growing groups of health care professionals, she noted. According to George, last year nearly 80,000 health care professionals pursued faculty development training; an adequate number of faculty is essential for training the next generation of health care workers. She further stated that almost 1.5 million health care professionals pursued continuing education; however, out of the nearly 9,000 continuing education courses that were offered, only 5 percent were specific to geriatric health care.

BARRIERS TO CARING FOR OLDER ADULTS

There are a number of barriers to increasing the supply of workers to care for the growing number of older adults, Hartley said. The pandemic had a dramatic impact on the workforce by exacerbating existing shortages. Pandemic-related employment losses in settings including hospitals and physicians' offices have largely recovered, while the losses in nursing care facilities and community care facilities have persisted (Figure 3-1).

Financial barriers can prevent individuals from pursuing jobs that involve caretaking of older adults, Hartley said. For example, the income of geriatricians in medicine is at or near the bottom of 30 medical specialties. For some, the cost of education may not be worth the earning potential. This disparity reflects systemic ageism, he said; society pays for what it values. Ageism is pervasive, particularly in Western cultures, and begins

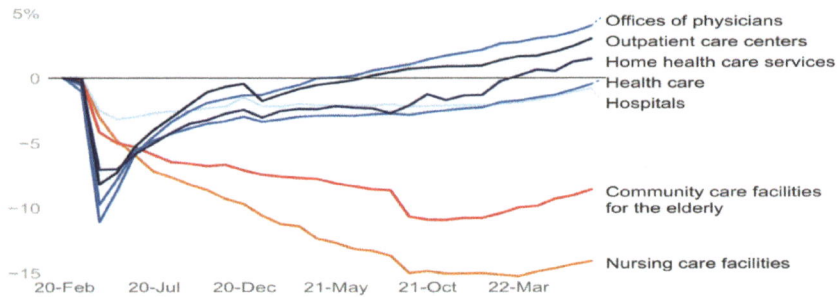

FIGURE 3-1 Pandemic-related employment losses in health care (cumulative percentage change in health sector employment by setting).
SOURCES: Hartley presentation, December 8, 2022; Wager, 2023, used with permission.

with "indoctrination" in early childhood that "aging is a bad thing." Messages embedded in nursery rhymes and fairy tales form attitudes and beliefs that infiltrate everything, including health care. Ageism affects health in two ways. First, it affects an individual's health outcomes and longevity; having a positive attitude about aging can extend life expectancy by as much as 7.5 years. Second, ageism among health care professionals can result in suboptimal care in a number of areas. For example, a patient's pain may be attributed to age alone, which can lead to a patient receiving inadequate treatment. A physical therapist may believe an older adult cannot lift heavier weights or perform more repetitions, resulting in slower improvement and worse outcomes. Professionals may hold implicit beliefs about the value and potential of older adults and make decisions such as placing an older adult in long-term care (instead of an alternative non-institutional setting). Clinical researchers have historically excluded older adults entirely from research studies (in particular, drug studies), though this has changed recently, he said. The World Health Organization has recognized ageism as a problem and created a campaign in 2021 to combat ageism and mitigate its harmful impacts. The Campaign to Combat Ageism includes social media posts, information in multiple languages, and powerful images (WHO, 2021).

Finally, there are barriers within health professions education that prevent students from pursuing careers in geriatrics. Most programs do not require a dedicated course in geriatrics, even though almost every health professional will work with this group at some point in their career. In contrast, he said, pediatrics is usually a required course despite the fact that only a fraction of providers will practice in this area. Around 42 percent of physical therapy programs offer a dedicated course in geriatrics. About

76 percent of medical schools provide an optional clinical experience in geriatrics, and 45 percent of programs require a geriatric rotation for all students (Dawson et al., 2022). Hartley posited that this inadequate attention to older adults stems in part from a belief that older adults are "just adults with more years of experience," instead of understanding that childhood, adulthood, and elderhood are three distinct phases of life (Aronson, 2019). He quoted a physician who said that most physicians graduate medical school lacking confidence in how to manage pain in a 90-year-old and that family practice doctors often know more about rare pediatric genetic diseases than they do about clearing an elderly patient for surgery.

Having grown up in a society full of messages that devalue older adults, students may be deterred from wanting to work in geriatrics or gerontology, Hartley said. Furthermore, implicit or explicit bias among faculty in health professions education programs can push students in other directions. For example, faculty may say or imply that caring for older adults is "boring," "depressing," or that "patients don't improve." Despite the growing population of older adults, the number of health care professionals focusing on geriatrics is actually declining, he said; for example, the number of first-year residents and fellows studying geriatrics declined by 14 percent between 2012 and 2017 (AAMC, 2018).

ROUNDTABLE DISCUSSION

With the presentations of George and Hartley in mind, the session turned to a roundtable discussion to explore the challenges of building an adequate workforce for older adults and to discuss potential solutions to these challenges. Hartley began by asking panelists what has inspired them, as well as the learners they work with, to pursue a career in working with older adults. Ryan Bradley, the director of research at the Helfgott Research Institute at the National University of Natural Medicine, responded that situational learning is vital to the clinical education experience. As a clinical educator of medical students and residents, he has observed that situational learning in primary care delivery to older adults has had a strong and positive impact on learners' interest in working with older adults in their careers. Bradley served as an attending physician in an integrative primary care clinic nested within a community-based senior center. His previous employer, Bastyr University, was invited to develop a clinic in this setting because the senior center leaders recognized that their community members had unmet needs, including highly uncoordinated care and a lack of guidance on nutrition, physical activity, and other approaches for improving function. Fourth-year medical students and residents at the clinic found their care delivery experience to be highly rewarding, Bradley said. The patients were appreciative of having care providers listen to their stories, coordinate their care, and give practical suggestions for improving their health. The trainees left the clinic each day challenged by the complexity of the care and also with a high degree of satisfaction because they felt they were really helping the older adults, he said.

He gave two examples of students whose experiences in the clinic influenced the direction of their careers. One student, after witnessing the need for dementia care, went on to operate a clinic that specializes exclusively in cognition care and also started a residential long-term care facility that incorporates many of the tenets of integrative medicine, including plant-based nutrition, combined cognitive and physical exercise, social support, and highly multidisciplinary care teams on site. Another student entered the clinic wanting to focus on traditional complementary medicine approaches (e.g., homeopathy, hydrotherapy). However, her experience in the senior care community clinic working with patients who had multiple chronic conditions and were taking multiple medicines, often without a provider managing their care, shifted her focus, and she now runs an integrative primary care clinic that focuses almost exclusively on older adults with multiple chronic conditions. Situational learning experiences like these are pivotal, Bradley said, both for students to learn about the considerable need that exists in this population and also to experience how rewarding it can be to work with "such an appreciative, responsive, and deserving group of people."

Lauren Mazzurco, a professor of geriatrics at Eastern Virginia Medical School, said she has had opportunities to work with learners across the continuum, from premed students to residents, fellows, and practitioners, and has used these opportunities to find out why they are interested in working with older adults. Many have had close relationships with older adults in their own lives and saw the frustrations and challenges that these adults had with their health care experiences. Learners are also motivated by the fact that geriatrics has one of the highest satisfaction rates of any medical specialty as well as by the focus on well-being, self-care, and quality of life. In geriatrics, she said, it is essential to not "miss the forest for the trees"; providers must look at every element of a patient's care and consider ways to improve function and independence. While taking care of an older adult can be "very overwhelming," Mazzurco said, job satisfaction and the ability to make a big impact can be surprising and empowering for learners. They take these lessons back to other specialties when on rotation, she said; for example, a surgery patient may have delirium, and the learner is better able to understand that individual's mental state and be more patient. The career paths for learners who wish to specialize in caring for older adults are currently quite limited, Mazzurco said, so she advocates for opening up more diverse specialty track pathways. However, regardless of what field learners pursue, their experiences with older adults can affect their future work and help to make health systems more age-friendly.

Working with older adults can be intimidating for new learners in health care, said Jeannine Lawrence, the senior associate dean in the Department of Human Nutrition at University of Alabama, particularly if the learner has not had any meaningful opportunities in his or her own life to interact with older adults in a positive manner. Learners often come into the profession with preconceived stereotypes about older adults; one of the challenges for educators is to break these stereotypes and show the diversity of the older adult population. Educators also need to enhance learners' intentions to and enthusiasm for working with older adults and increase their confidence and skills in doing so. In nutrition—and other health fields—one significant predictor of intentions to work with older adults is attitudes toward older adults. Providing frequent and quality interactions with older adults in a variety of settings is very effective at positively affecting learner attitudes towards working with older adults, Lawrence said. She explained that this means that students need more than a single rotation in a long-term care facility; they also need other opportunities to engage with older adults, such as through partnerships with community agencies or working with seniors who live independently. Subjective norms provide another strong predictor of intentions to work with older adults. When faculty and other role models themselves work with and talk about older adults, it can create a perception that this is a valuable career path and inspire learners to follow such a path. Finally, Lawrence said, learners need interprofessional education and training to prepare themselves for geriatric practice; it can be a real deterrent to students who think they will be solely responsible for making decisions about the complex care of older adults.

Lawrence told workshop participants about a program she and her colleagues developed to address confidence and roles in a health care team. Nutrition, nursing, social work, and medical students sat together and discussed their scope of practice and perceived roles within the team; Lawrence said it was "pretty fun" because none of the students had any idea what training or skills the other students had. The teams then went out and worked with rural older adults over a period of 6 months to assess and address their health care and daily living needs. During this time, the students experienced a rapid upturn in confidence in both working and connecting with the older adult participants, as well as building reliance and trust in their own team. The students no longer felt unprepared to meet the needs of the 38 participants because they knew exactly who on the team to turn to when a need was identified. After this experience, the students reported feeling more confident working with older adults and with other health care professionals. Encouraging and inspiring learners to work with older adults requires a multi-pronged approach, Lawrence said, including providing high-quality interactions with older adults, varied and regular experiences, good role models, and interprofessional training.

Financial Barriers

Hartley next turned to financial barriers. He asked Rajean Moone, the faculty director for long-term care administration in the College of Continuing and Professional Studies at the University of Minnesota, to comment on incentive structures for encouraging health care students and professionals to work with older adults. "We don't have long lines of students entering gerontological and geriatric practice," Moone said, so incentives—particularly financial incentives—are important to the efforts to increase the workforce and improve senior care. However, he continued, they are often seen as a panacea that will magically solve all of the problems. In practice, the success of financial incentives is contingent upon other systemic factors and reform. Incentives are fairly straightforward and are not a new phenomenon; the basic principle is that humans are driven toward rewards and away from negative experiences. Incentives in the senior care workforce tend to be a patchwork of state and federal programs, and they are often under-resourced.

Financial incentives can fall into several categories. The first are incentives for students currently in school. These could include scholarship programs and paid internships working with older adults. The second is incentives for those who have already graduated. Loan forgiveness is paramount in this area, and many states have piloted and implemented loan-forgiveness programs for those who work in senior care, particularly in rural and other underserved areas. The third type of incentive is for those already working in senior care, such as increased wages or competitive benefits. Moone warned, however, that wages and benefits are part of a much larger and more complicated conversation about long-term care financing reform. The nursing home sector has suffered for decades from underinvestment and a lack of accountability in how resources are allocated. In Minnesota, he said, the average hourly wage for a direct-care staff member in senior care is around $16 per hour; in comparison, the starting hourly wage at a major retailer is $20 per hour with full benefits and tuition assistance. There were a few incentives that were implemented during COVID—primarily relaxing barriers to certifications and credentials—that are being phased out. These have provided a temporary boost to the senior care workforce, but the impact on the quality of care is unclear.

Unfortunately, there is not a great deal of longitudinal literature of the effectiveness of financial incentives aimed at students, recent graduates, or workers. It is clear that incentives can provide a temporary boost, but their long-term sustainability is not clear. Moone said that there are larger-scale, systemic changes that have the potential for increasing the workforce, such as immigration reform or increasing reimbursement rates, but these are not often considered in conversations about workforce incentives. There

Incentivizing Nurses

Hartley asked Barbara Resnick, a professor in the Department of Organizational Systems and Adult Health at the University of Maryland School of Nursing, for her perspective on non-financial incentives that could encourage people to choose careers working with older adults. Resnick responded that the conversation about a looming boom of older adults and the lack of an adequate health care workforce often "dances around what needs to be done." She put it bluntly: "Change the law, and you change behavior." All people working in health care are going to be dealing with older adults in some way, she said, and they should be required to learn about this population. In nursing, every adult nurse practitioner is required to be trained in geriatric care. This needs to be done across all health disciplines, Resnick said; this is the "number one way to change things." Once exposed to working with older adults, there will be some learners who realize how much they enjoy the field. For others, they will simply be trained in how to better care for older adults across all settings. After all, she commented, even in pediatrics one has to care for and address the grandparents. A second way, as many other speakers have noted, is to expose students to older adults. However, educators have the responsibility to make these experiences fun and opportunities for learning critically important assessment, diagnosis, and management skills, rather than presenting long-term care as a "negative, horrible clinical experience." The third approach for encouraging students to work with older adults is to focus on job opportunities and job security. Resnick said that she tells her students that the best positions are in long-term care because they will see diseases and have experiences they would not have otherwise, they will have a team to work with, and they will be able to change how care is provided. Resnick agreed with Moone that incentives are often a short-term fix and that structural changes are needed to truly improve the system.

Specialization Issues

In medicine, geriatrics is usually a sub-specialty of internal medicine or family medicine, Hartley said. Other professions have also created specialties or sub-specialties for working with older adults, but it can be a struggle to get people to choose these specialties. Hartley asked panelists to comment on this challenge. Mazzurco said that this is a big problem and that there need to be creative solutions. She noted that while there is "big G geriatrics" (highly trained board-certified geriatricians of which the numbers are dwindling), there is also "little g geriatrics" (geriatric scholars who teach geriatrics principles to all health professions and to the public), and both are important (Callahan et al., 2017). The American Geriatric Society has made some innovative efforts in this area, such as integrated residencies and fellowships; this allows learners to gain experience in geriatrics from the very beginning of residency rather than waiting until the end to do specialty training. Some providers who are already practicing and have realized the gap in their own knowledge and skill set in caring for older adults may wish to pursue a geriatrics fellowship, Mazzurco said, but it is just not logistically possible for many people. There are innovative models evolving that offer fellowships that fit within providers' lives, such as "interrupted fellowships" that allow providers to work in between rotations for the fellowship. Until geriatrics training is required for all health professions learners, these types of programs can bridge the gap and provide creative solutions for training people in geriatrics.

George added that in addition to the challenge of getting learners to specialize in geriatric care, primary care as a specialty is undervalued in medicine. This will have a big impact on the older adult population moving forward, she said. Learners come out of medical education with hundreds of thousands of dollars of debt, and they are not incentivized to enter a field that will make it challenging to pay off their debt.

Role of Families and Lay Caregivers

Given the likely inadequate workforce and the growing older adult population, Hartley said, much of the care of older adults will be provided by lay people and untrained individuals. Hartley asked panelists for thoughts on how these caregivers could potentially be trained or integrated into the health system. Resnick responded that there is a big initiative in nursing to conduct family trainings; she said that "the expectations now on families are mind boggling." Nurses often are the ones who most closely interact with families, particularly during transitions of care. Nurses need training in cultural competence, communication, and other skills to help them reach these families. Resnick said there are opportunities to bring families into acute or subacute care environments to allow them to begin to practice the skills they will need at home, noting that as a mother of triplets in the neonatal intensive care unit, she insisted on providing as much care as she could to her babies. Another way to train lay people, she said, is with apprenticeship programs, which were historically very common in medicine and nursing.

Bradley said that while family members can play a very important role, "we need to be really careful to not redirect the responsibility of health care back to family members." The responsibility of primary care is to help patients navigate their care and develop coordinated care plans, and this should not be placed on the shoulders of family members. There are other professionals who could be used, such as health coaches, who could contribute to senior care if they were empowered to serve in this role. Family members are important for patient care, but the health care delivery system and community still holds primary responsibility in this regard. Maryam Tabrizi, a geriatric dentist at the University of Nevada Las Vegas agreed with Bradley, saying that care providers open the "door to neglect" when they pass the responsibility for care to family members. Caring for older adults is exhausting and can last years, she said, and the emotions involved can make it even more challenging.

Role of State Policy

Shirley Girouard, who is part of the nursing faculty at the State University of New York Downstate, asked about state policies that could be helpful in expanding and strengthening the workforce for older adult care. Moone replied that many incentives, particularly financial incentives, are the product of state legislation, and states can also choose to relax requirements for certification and credentials. In addition, states have key roles in broader workforce development. In Minnesota, for example, there is currently a huge number of open positions in senior care, and many senior care communities have to deny admission because they do not have enough workers to care for people. With record unemployment rates and competition from other employers, it is time to have a complex conversation about changing the way that long-term care is financed. In particular, he explained, a key issue is paying for the real value of nurses. Any conversation about this will require confronting difficult topics such as sexism and racism and the value that society places on different members of our communities.

Hartley pointed out the need for macro, meso, and micro levels of change. At the micro level, there is a need to advocate for changes in accreditation standards and require geriatrics for all learners. At the meso level, there is a need to advocate for state legislators to do their part to bolster the workforce. At the macro level, federal action on the financing of long-term care or long-term support services is needed, along with discussions about Medicare and Medicaid payments.

Defining Quality

Bradley noted that several speakers during the workshop had brought up the issue of not sacrificing quality when considering innovations in training and care delivery. Quality is of course essential, he said, but he urged stakeholders to consider what quality means to the older adults themselves. Within the health professions, quality is sometimes defined by process metrics or processes, but patients are looking for things that improve their quality of life, function, and health. He emphasized the need to think outside the box about what really matters to the individual and to keep the focus on that.

4

Addressing the Gap

Key Messages Made by Presenters

- Opportunities for students are not available at all institutions, and students are not always inclined to voluntarily learn about older adults. (Brickman)
- The Dementia Friends program resulted in statistically improved attitudes among students about persons with dementia. (McCarthy)
- Age-friendly universities use a framework of ten principles that relate to the active engagement of older adults in campus life. (Moone)
- The Virtual Interprofessional Consultation Clinic sessions consist of an introduction to the process, multiple 5- to 8-minute patient assessments, and questions, followed by an interprofessional discussion and development of the clinical assessment note by the students/trainees without the patient present. (Hicks-Roof)

With a rapidly growing population of older adults, there is a pressing demand to expand and strengthen the workforce of health professionals caring for older adults. However, there are a number of challenges in doing so, including ageism, lack of opportunities to engage with older adults, and a lack of interest among many health professionals in working with older adult populations. In this workshop session, speakers presented details about innovative programs and initiatives that are addressing these challenges and building a strong health care workforce for older adults.

CHANGING ATTITUDES ABOUT WORKING WITH OLDER ADULTS

Lily Brickman, a recent graduate of the master's program in food science and human nutrition at the University of Maine, spoke to workshop participants about her experience as a dietetic student working with older adults. Brickman said she had always wanted to be a dietitian and that after working in a nursing home she began to realize the importance of proper nutrition for older adults. In graduate school, she was given the opportunity to work as a graduate assistant under the Geriatric Workforce Enhancement Program. Part of her responsibilities was helping out with a course at the University of Maine on nutritional care for older adults. Brickman said that only four or five students enrolled in the course each semester that she worked on the course and that in the past semester no students were registered. After talking with her thesis advisor, Brickman decided to focus her masters' thesis research on educating dietetic students about the nutritional concerns of older adults. The goals of her research were to examine the interest of dietetics students in working with older adults and to understand different academic programs' needs for teaching dietetics students in this area. Brickman conducted two surveys, one of the food science and human nutrition students at University of Maine and another of the Nutrition and Dietetic Educators and Preceptors (NDEP) group, an organizational unit of the Academy of Nutrition Dietetics. NDEP consists of a wide variety of professionals, Brickman said, including educators, faculty, internship directors, internship preceptors, and program coordinators. The response rate to her surveys was low, she said, but there were still valuable insights gained.

Given the expected growth in the older adult population, the availability of opportunities for dietetics students to learn about older adults must be increased, Brickman said. Opportunities for students are not available at all institutions, and students are not always inclined to voluntarily learn about older adults. If offering full courses is not feasible, relevant content should be added into existing courses. It is also critical, she said, to educate credentialed dietitians and other nutrition professionals about nutrition in older adults and provide incentives such as continuing education credits. Registered dietitians need 15 continuing education credits each year; this is a great opportunity to reach these professionals, she said. Brickman expressed her hope that her research provides insight into student interest in learning and working with older adults as well as insight into the availability of older adult nutrition education at institutions across the United States. She emphasized that further research is needed regarding effective strategies for increasing student interest in working with older adults.

Jeannine Lawrence from the University of Alabama asked Brickman to reflect on her learning opportunities in the area of nutrition and older adults and on what worked best for her as a learner. Brickman responded that in her nutrition/geriatrics classes, what was most beneficial were hands-on activities that allowed students to interview and speak with older adults about their health, their lifestyle, and what changes needed to be made. In the literature she reviewed for her thesis, Brickman said, research indicated that these types of hands-on experiences can improve health professions students' interest in and attitude toward working with older adults; these experiences could include performing exams, using a simulation, or working with older adults on their mobility challenges. Such activities, Brickman said, are effective ways for students to gain an understanding of the challenges that older adults face and to change learner attitudes about working with this population. George, also a student, agreed that direct experience—with any population—is what often leads to interest in working in a particular area. Hazen said that as a nursing doctoral student, she had observed that Brickman herself became interested in working with older adults based on her personal experiences working in nursing homes. George said that older adults are often not particularly visible in our society, so opportunities to interact with older adults need to be made more readily available. Intergenerational relationships can be rich and meaningful, and not having the opportunity to build these relationships is a "huge loss" for everyone, George said. In addition, content about healthy aging needs to be integrated early and often into health professions education programs. George said that she is in her last year of medical school and has yet to take a course on healthy aging. She is currently developing a course herself; she said that it is essential for people who are passionate in this area to take actions that force changes. The course she is developing will be required, which she said is important because people often do not know what they are interested in until they learn more about it. Annette Greer, a researcher in interprofessional education at East Carolina University, noted that health professions curricula are often driven by what is on the licensing exam. If there are few or no questions about aging on an exam, the topic is unlikely to be covered in a curriculum. There is a need for national boards to value this population and to acknowledge that older adults are a population for which caregivers need specific education and training.

Katie Eliot of the Department of Nutritional Sciences at The University of Oklahoma Health Sciences Center asked Brickman and George to comment on the role of faculty and how they can serve as role models for students making decisions about career paths. Brickman responded that the faculty members at her school often share stories about their work—whether in community nutrition, clinical nutrition, or other areas—and about the impact their work has had on patients or community members. These stories, she said, are inspirational and have made her more certain about her career. George added that her focus is on palliative care and that many of her early mentors were palliative care physicians who emphasized the humanity of patients and the importance of relationship. Once she began medical school, she said, she found that the focus was often on pathology rather than personhood. However, George said that she felt lucky to have found some faculty mentors centered on the human being rather than the disease. This is a major issue both in health professions education and in practice, she said, particularly among older adults who can feel that providers are focusing on their diseases rather than on them as individual people. Just as learners need exposure to older adults to know if they want to work in that area, George said, learners also need mentors to show them what is possible and to open their eyes to new perspectives.

ATTITUDES ABOUT MEMORY LOSS

Teresa McCarthy, a geriatrician and associate professor of medicine in the Department of Family Medicine at the University of Minnesota, and Teresa Schicker, a program manager of the Minnesota Northstar Geriatric Workforce Enhancement Program at the University of Minnesota, told workshop participants about a simple, effective intervention to increase awareness of dementia, and they explored how activities such as this could impact the future workforce. McCarthy said that as a clinical educator, she has been teaching geriatrics for many years to students from many health professions. Because more students have been required to participate in geriatrics rotations in recent years, she learned that many trainees have had absolutely no exposure to older people or dementia. She also uncovered a lot of misperceptions and ageism in the trainee group as well as a lack of empathy. McCarthy said she looked for a module or activity she could use to address this problem, and she came across the Dementia Friends program. This is a worldwide movement to develop age-friendly and dementia-friendly communities. The core component of the program, she said, is information sessions that use a "train the trainer" model; people who attend sessions can take a brief training and then take the content into their own communities. It is explicitly not an education session, McCarthy emphasized, but rather an information session by community members to community members. It consists of 60 minutes of scripted content that is proprietary but free to access. Sessions can be held in person or virtually, with up to 70 participants. The session focuses on five key messages about dementia:

- Dementia is not a normal part of aging;
- Dementia is caused by diseases of the brain;
- Dementia is not just about having memory problems;
- It is possible to have good quality of life with dementia;
- There is more to a person than his or her dementia.

Content is delivered in an "upbeat" and "comfortable" way, she said, with some individual activities to reflect on one's perspectives on aging and dementia. Small group interactions and story telling allow the trainers to augment the content with their own life experiences, which really enhances the experience for learners. At the end, there are practical recommendations for effective communication with people with Alzheimer's disease. McCarthy said that residents find the content interesting and helpful.

McCarthy showed an image that is used in the Dementia Friends training (Figure 4-1). The image is of two bookcases, one representing the healthy brain and one representing the brain of a person with progressing dementia. The bookshelf of the dementia patient has been "shaken," which results in many of the books on the top falling off; these are analogous to facts and complex thinking. However, most of the books on the bottom stay

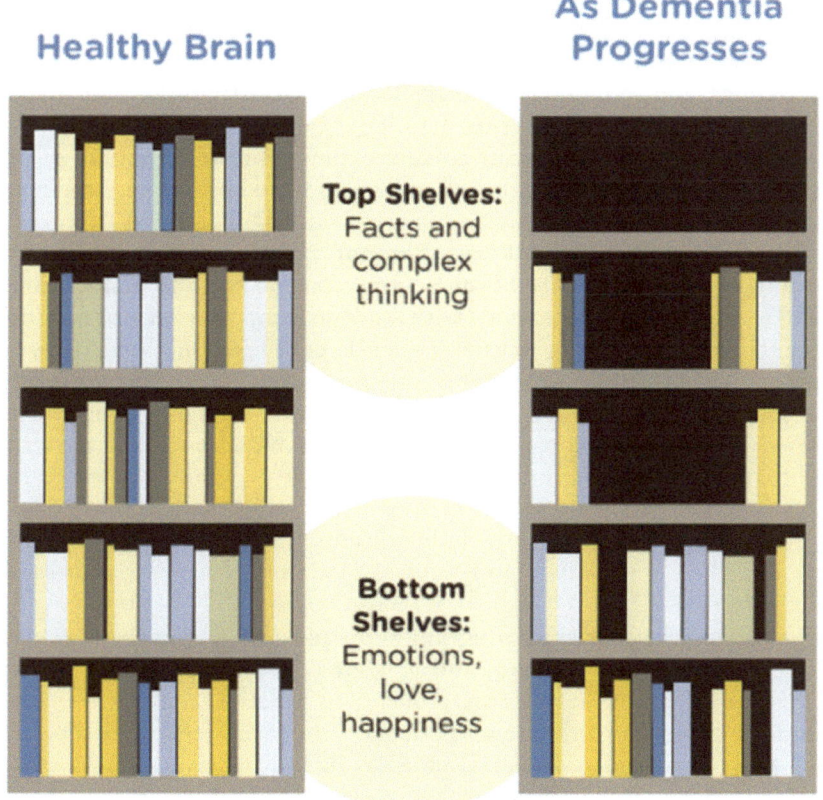

FIGURE 4-1 Bookcase analogy from Dementia Friends.
SOURCE: McCarthy presentation, December 8, 2022.

in place when shaken; these books are analogous to emotions, love, and sense of self. This is a great visual for understanding dementia, McCarthy said, and it provides context for how to interact with dementia patients.

McCarthy said that she used the Dementia Friends program with her students and wanted to evaluate what impact it was having on their attitudes and knowledge. She and her colleagues and students developed a study that surveyed around 100 students (medical, physical therapy, and pharmacy) before and after the program. The study used a validated 20-question scale called the Dementia Attitudes Scale (O'Connor and McFadden, 2010), which incorporates both knowledge about these diseases as well as a person's comfort in interacting with dementia patients. The study found that the program resulted in statistically improved attitudes. The takeaway message, McCarthy said, is that a modest effort information session, delivered by students and lay people, increased knowledge and improved attitudes of health professional students towards those living with dementia.

Schicker provided details about how the Dementia Friends program was implemented at the University of Minnesota. She said that the program can be implemented in a variety of settings, including academic institutions, clinical settings, and community settings. Because of the train-the-trainer model, there have been several students who have "taken it and run with it," she said. For example, a pharmacy student expanded it to the school of pharmacy, and several of that student's colleagues have become trainers in turn. This is an excellent opportunity, Shicker said, for leadership development among health professions students. Thus far at the University of Minnesota, the program has trained 164 health professionals and community members and 825 health science students, with students coming from areas including nursing, physical therapy, mortuary science, education and human development, and public health. Next year, the program will be offered at primary care clinics around the state. Schicker stressed that Dementia Friends can be offered in informal settings such as student clubs, libraries, or classrooms and that it can be done online or in person. The program is proprietary, so it must be licensed through the U.S. or U.K. branch of Dementia Friends. Schicker urged stakeholders to hold sessions for interprofessional groups, although she noted that offering classes made up of a single profession is also an option.

The Dementia Friends program is a "pleasant experience for everybody involved," Shicker said, and it is effective and building knowledge and empathy. Health professions students or practitioners can also recommend the program to their own patients or to caregivers of their patients. McCarthy commented on how Dementia Friends received some pushback early on from health professions faculty because the program presents very basic information and does not "dig deep" into pathology. However, the reason that the program resonates is its "gut impact," which augments the underlying content, as well as the way it provides an understanding of what it is like to live with dementia.

AGE-FRIENDLY UNIVERSITIES

There are a variety of age-friendly initiatives in a number of sectors, Rajean Moone said. For example, the World Health Organization and AARP have a framework for age-friendly communities, which allows people to assess a community and look for opportunities for a community to become more age-friendly. There are also efforts in the area of health systems, public health, businesses, creativity and the arts, and universities. All of these efforts come together under the umbrella of an age-friendly ecosystem; Moone said that institutions following age-friendly principles are making a commitment to the future and to moving the needle toward a more inclusive, supportive environment for an aging population. He also shared details about age-friendly universities and the principles that guide them. Age-friendly universities use a framework of 10 principles in areas that include online educational opportunities, a range of educational needs, health and wellness, research agenda, and second careers. All of these principles, he said, relate to the active engagement of older adults in campus life. One of the 10 principles, intergenerational learning, is aimed at facilitating the reciprocal sharing of expertise among learners of all ages. Intergenerational learning has a number of benefits, including exposing younger students to older adults and affecting their attitudes and beliefs about age and potential career paths.

To begin the process of helping the University of Minnesota (UMN) become an age-friendly university, a task force was created that was made up of individuals representing programs incentivized to work with older adults across campus. The task force started by sharing information. Moone explained that UMN is an enormous campus, so people are often siloed in their own areas. The task force enabled collaborative work across siloes. The task force conducted an assessment that looked at all departments and services, including arts, sports, enrollment, and employment. UMN used a tool created by the University of Massachusetts to inventory all programs and services and identify opportunities to build capacity. After the results of the assessment were presented to university leadership, the university president formed the Age-Friendly University of Minnesota Council and enrolled UMN in the global network.[1] Enrollment in the network was the "easiest part" of the process, Moone said; the hardest part was finding the resources

---

[1] The Age-Friendly University (AFU) global network is made up of institutions of higher education from around the world that have endorsed and acted upon the 10 AFU principles (Gerontological Society of America, 2023).

and time required to fully examine the university's age-friendliness and making a commitment to change.

The UMN council is made up of a number of entities across campus, including the Alumni Association, the Women's Club, the Office of Public Engagement, the Center for Healthy Aging and Innovation, the Osher Lifelong Learning Institution, the MN Northstar Geriatrics Workforce Enhancement Program, and the Retirees' Association. Critical to the success of the program were community partnerships, Moone said. He is an appointed member of the Governor's Council for an Age-Friendly Minnesota, which allows him to bring the university lens to the broader conversation about age-friendliness in the state. Community partnerships with UMN include partnerships with the state unit on aging health systems, area agencies on aging, home- and community-based service providers, AARP, senior housing, and the media. Moone said that one of the first major activities of the UMN Age-Friendly Council was establishing Age-Friendly University Day, which was dedicated to bringing life-long learners, retirees, and older Minnesotans to campus to converse about various topics relevant to their lives and to get them accustomed to coming to campus. There was a fireside chat with a former Minnesota Supreme Court justice and another with a former Minnesota Vikings player; these events excited and attracted older adults, Moone said. Media are a critical partner in these efforts, he said, for telling the story and getting the word out about the activities and initiatives at the university.

Moone asked breakout room participants to share questions or comments about their own experiences. Eliot commented that as a registered dietitian, she thinks about the way food systems and nutrition interact with the aging population. She asked Moone if the age-friendly initiatives at UMN involve this area. He responded that the Center for Nutrition Studies at UMN has largely been focused on nutrition in early life. However, the center has also been exploring the issue of food insecurity and older adults. UMN, in conjunction with the state, has been looking at rates of participation in the Supplemental Nutrition Assistance Program and has found that the rate of uptake in seniors is quite low compared with other populations. In response to this finding, the center has done targeted outreach to these communities. Moone said that his own lens on nutrition is quite different; he focuses on long-term care administrators and looks at innovations in nutrition (e.g., research on making food more appealing).

A workshop participant, Delfina Alvarez, asked Moone to comment on whether there is any collaboration or coordination between the age-friendly university network and the age-friendly community network. He responded by sharing one example of such collaboration. At the Age-Friendly University Day, AARP put on a presentation about age-friendly communities and gave people information about how they can get involved in these efforts.

Another way in which these two entities collaborate is by having a representative from the university help out when a community is undergoing the process of becoming age-friendly. For example, it can be helpful to have an academic voice present evidence to policy makers in discussions about allocating resources to age-friendly community initiatives.

Patrick DeLeon, a psychologist professor with the Uniformed Services University of the Health Sciences, asked Moone how to institutionalize age-friendliness into universities rather than relying on the passion and dedication of individual faculty members. DeLeon noted that good ideas can easily come and go, depending on what the next generation of leaders wants to do. Moone responded that this is always a major consideration for him and that a key first step was getting the president to appoint an official council. This is now part of the university makeup, with bylaws to formalize the work. While bylaws can pigeonhole and restrain some efforts, they also contribute to stability and sustainability. The other consideration for sustainability, he said, is ensuring that there are resources available and processes in place to continue efforts when dedicated leaders leave. There is no magic answer, Moone said, but the most sustainable programs are those that rely on a collaborative of people rather than on a few individuals.

Kim Dunleavy with the Department of Physical Therapy at the University of Florida and representing the American Council of Academic Physical Therapy mentioned that her institution's program pairs students with older adults in the community, which can lead to instances of ageism and mismatched expectations. Students are keen to help the adults with specific projects around their homes, she said, but they often do not see the social component as important. Jacqueline Kreinik, a nurse and subject matter expert at the Centers for Medicare & Medicaid Services, said that the first stage of working with older adults is listening. Students need to set aside their expectations and focus on what matters most for the older adults. Health professions students, as well as practitioners, often want to jump in and make big changes to "be a hero," but the older adult may want the person to simply listen or to lend a helping hand.

Maxwell described a program at her institution called Frailty-Focused Communication (Maxwell et al., 2022). Within this program, a workshop gives students a more in-depth understanding of the process of ageing, and there is a focus on communicating with older adults and using motivational interviewing skills to discuss issues deemed important by this population. Students are paired with an older adult in the community and then encouraged to develop a relationship and a friendship. A recent publication gives details on the program (Miller et al., 2022). Following up on Maxwell's remarks, Jennifer Cabrera, a workshop participant, agreed that communication can be difficult between younger students or residents and older adults. She noted that older adults can get "left behind" because they cannot keep up with the pace and that getting younger residents to sit and listen to an older patient for a few minutes can be a real challenge. Moone responded by saying that a pivotal part of his experience was going to undergraduate school on a campus with a nursing home. Most students volunteered or worked at the home at some point, and being able to build relationships, relate to other people, and build empathy are part of the critical "soft skills" of education. The pinnacle of geriatrics, Moone said, is helping health professions students build these types of critical skills so that they are able to listen to their patients and discover what matters.

VIRTUAL INTERPROFESSIONAL CONSULTATION CLINIC

Kristen Hicks-Roof, an associate professor in the Department of Nutrition and Dietetics at the University of North Florida, told participants about how she and her colleagues developed the Virtual Interprofessional (VIP) Consultation Clinic. It began, she said, with an interprofessional education series (IPES), which consisted of discussion and education sessions that focused on topics including communication, role responsibility, and team-based care. Participants included physical therapy residents, occupational therapy residents, family medicine residents, and dietetic interns; they met in a virtual environment in the years before this became common during COVID-19. IPES used hypothetical case examples to guide discussions, Hicks-Roof said, but numerous trainees participants requested real-life interactions with patients. Based on this and other feedback, the VIP Consultation Clinic was developed.

The VIP experience (Figure 4-2) begins with an orientation session focusing on roles and responsibilities. Hicks-Roof described research showing that if health professionals are not aware of what other health professionals actually do, they are less likely to refer patients to them or work together. In the orientation participants are taught about who other health professionals are, how they are educated, and where and how they work. This facilitates greater understanding and respect among the group, she said. After orientation, groups of learners participate in VIP sessions with patients. These sessions consist of an introduction to the process, multiple 5- to 8-minute patient assessments, and questions, followed by an interprofessional discussion and development of the clinical assessment notes without the patient present. Participating residents are from a range of disciplines, including physical therapy, occupational therapy, family medicine, nursing (D.N.P.), dietetics, and clinical mental health counseling. Patients are usually referred, and they are paid $75 for their participation. The program does not specifically recruit older adults as patients, but many participants are older, she said.

VIP participants are surveyed after the conclusion of the program, and Hicks-Roof presented several findings based on these surveys. First, there

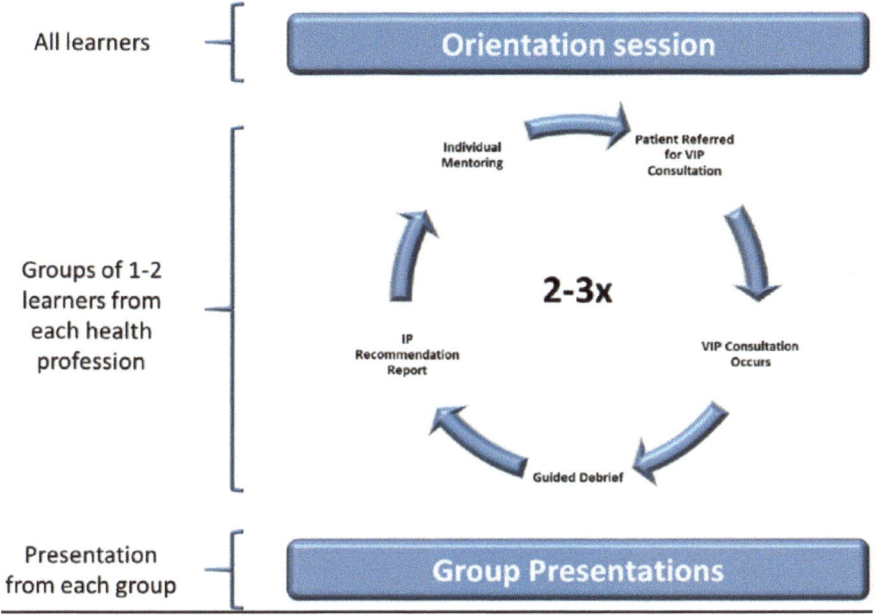

FIGURE 4-2 Virtual Interprofessional (VIP) Consultation Clinic learning model.
SOURCE: Hicks-Roof presentation, December 8, 2022.

is a strong perceived positive impact on future interprofessional collaborative practice (Figure 4-3). This impact is particularly strong among mental health counselors and registered dietitians; Hicks-Roof noted that these two groups are newer to the world of interprofessional training. Second, most participants were more likely to refer to the other professions after the program than before. Again, the impact was greatest in the areas of nutrition and mental health, which Hicks-Roof noted are of critical importance for the health of older adults.

There were many advantages of the VIP clinic program, Hicks-Roof said. Learners have an opportunity to train on virtual technology and telehealth delivery and are exposed to older adults. Learners can participate in real patient assessments and are able to discuss and reflect on the assessments with an inclusive group of professionals. At the same time, the patients gain access to a wide variety of expertise in one clinic visit, which is quite uncommon. The program can be integrated into resident and intern schedules and competencies, Hicks-Roof said. The challenges associated with the program include recruitment of patients, scheduling VIP consults, ensuring continuous care for patients, and technical issues in the virtual

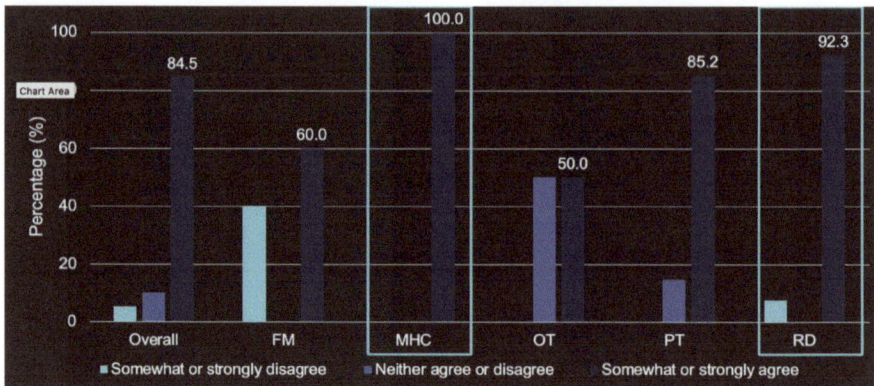

FIGURE 4-3 Virtual Interprofessional (VIP) Consultation Clinic's perceived positive impact on future interprofessional collaboration.
SOURCE: Hicks-Roof presentation, December 8, 2022.

environment. The technical issues are a particular problem when working with older adults, she said, who sometimes have more trouble navigating virtual visits.

Hicks-Roof asked breakout group participants to share their thoughts and questions. Greer asked how learner competencies and patient health outcomes are measured. Hicks-Roof responded that learners are given pre- and post-surveys with both quantitative and qualitative measures. Patients participate in only two VIP clinics, so there is less information gathered on them and their experience. Hicks-Roof said it would be helpful to follow patients over a longer period to see whether and how the experience affects their care. She posited that one benefit of participation for patients is simply exposure to other types of health professionals, and she suggested that patients may in the future ask their primary providers for referrals based on their experiences. Kolasa added that this exposure goes both ways—health professionals participating in the VIP clinic gain exposure to older adults and get experience caring for this population. Greer commented that the National Academies of Practice has developed interprofessional telehealth competencies; these would be useful for measuring the impact of the VIP program for learners, she said. In addition, she suggested that integrating the VIP clinic with a patient's primary care provider could make it possible to track metrics and health outcomes (e.g., if a patient's diabetes markers improve after participation). Hicks-Roof agreed with Greer's concerns and said that a long-term vision is to create an embedded hybrid clinic within the family medicine residency program, which could address the concerns about measuring and tracking patient health outcomes.

Hartley noted that the VIP program is grant-funded and asked Hicks-Roof to comment on the value and sustainability of the program. Hicks-Roof responded that part of the reason for hoping to move to an embedded clinic in the family medicine program is to ensure the sustainability of the program. The idea, she said, would be for patients to be seen in person by family medicine practitioners in addition to participating in an interdisciplinary virtual session with other professionals. This could help with the continuity of care for patients as well as with sustainability. Hartley said that integrating the program into an existing care program could also potentially help with the reproducibility and scalability of the VIP program. Nina Tomasa, a workshop participant, closed the session by emphasizing that patients are an integral part of the care team and that the VIP model ideally welcomes patients in as part of the interprofessional collaboration.

CONTINUING PROFESSIONAL DEVELOPMENT IN GERIATRIC CARE

Josea Kramer, the associate director for education/evaluation of the geriatric research, education and clinical center (GRECC) at the Department of Veterans Affairs (VA) Greater Los Angeles Healthcare System, said that GRECCs are congressionally mandated centers of excellence that were established in the mid 1970s to meet the emerging "age wave" of older veterans by advancing geriatrics and gerontology. Each of the 20 GRECCs has a wide portfolio of clinical and research activities; the education component includes clinical training and fellowships across a variety of health professions as well as continuing education.

Kramer began the Geriatric Scholars Program in 2008 in response to the IOM report *Retooling for an Aging America,* which emphasized the importance of training the workforce that is already in place (IOM, 2008). The program is grant-funded by the VA Office of Rural Health and VA Office of Geriatrics and Extended Care.

The Geriatric Scholars Program was developed with a focus on the general primary care setting where most older veterans receive health care. The pilot program enrolled only primary care providers and expanded to additional disciplines within the medical home model of primary care, including pharmacists, psychologists, social workers, rehabilitation therapists, and psychiatrists. This national workforce development program evolved over the years into its current structure (Figure 4-4) of five integrated components, Kramer said. The core component focuses on individual clinicians who receive an intensive didactic program in geriatrics and gerontology along with an intensive workshop in quality improvement. Each participant initiates a quality improvement project in his or her own local setting. The quality improvement component gives participants an opportunity to

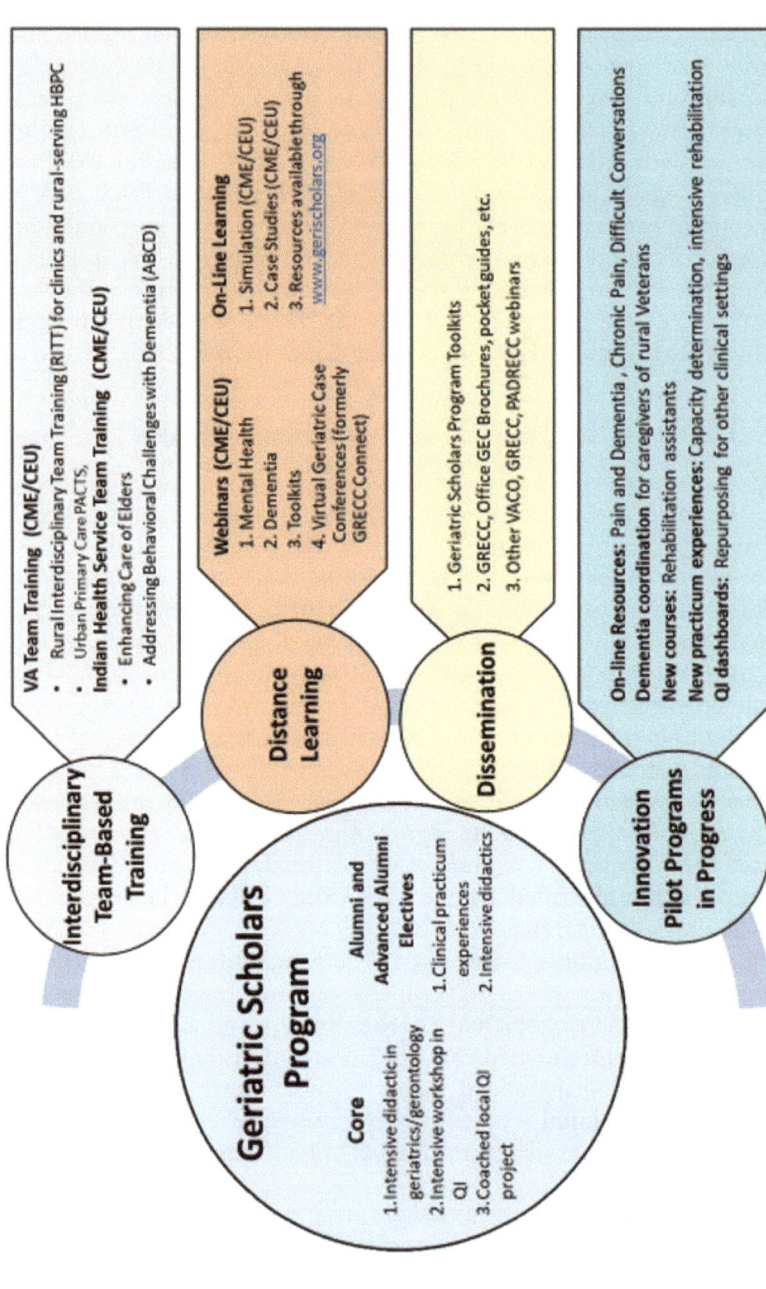

FIGURE 4-4 Geriatric Scholars Program.
SOURCE: Kramer presentation, December 8, 2022.

become "ambassadors for change," Kramer said, and provides "stealth education" in teaching new knowledge to the local clinical team in implementing quality improvement. One unique aspect is the longitudinal design for continuing education. The program is a longitudinal effort; after completing this program, there are opportunities for alumni to continue additional training and improve their skills over time. Immediately following the training, at 6 months post-training, and then at intervals thereafter, program participants are asked to self-identify learning gaps and additional topics of interest for future training. Using this information, Kramer said, new continuing education programs are developed annually; about 50 continuing education programs are offered each year.

Other unique aspects are the range of continuing education training opportunities across a number of health care professions; most are accredited as continuing medical education (CME) for VA and for non-VA participants and are awarded continuing education units (CEUs). In addition to training individual scholars, this national training program is intended to improve geriatric care through interdisciplinary team-based training, distance learning, dissemination, and pilot programs. Team-based training teaches everyone in the clinic—lay and professional clinical staff—to recognize common problems among older adults that may require immediate attention during the clinical visit, to implement team-based solutions to care, and to improve clinic efficiency. This component supports each discipline's critical role in patient interaction and making a difference in patients' care. Team training is offered to rural VA and Indian Health Service clinics as well as to urban VA primary care teams. Distance learning efforts include webinars, on-line resources, and simulations on such topics as dementia and mental health; most of these programs are accredited for CME/CEU for VA and for non-VA participants. The program's innovation arm develops and tests new educational programs; successful curricula are integrated into the regular program offerings and new resources, and tools that prove beneficial are disseminated. Around 1,400 scholars have completed the core Geriatric Scholars Program, and about 7,500 individuals have been reached through the team-based training and distance learning efforts, Kramer said.

Kramer described some lessons learned from the Geriatric Scholars Program. Being nimble and innovating quickly is critical, she said, and it is important to avoid mission drift. The longitudinal model can be adapted or adopted in other health systems. For example, the Indian Health Service is currently implementing its version of the Geriatric Scholars Program to meet a need to enhance geriatric expertise across its national health care system.

Martin MacDowell, a workshop participant, asked Kramer about how wellness and health promotion fit into the Geriatric Scholars Program. So many of the health issues of older adults, he said, are avoidable if people receive accurate and timely information about improving their health. Kramer responded that the VA has a strong emphasis on whole health and integrated health and that while this is not a major focus of the Geriatric Scholars Program, it is part of the overall environment and is included in many aspects of the program. Another workshop participant, Jennifer Cabrera, followed up on this by saying that the physical therapy department is often underused in this population and that physical therapists can be a great resource for helping older adults stay active and healthy. Physical therapy is often an "afterthought" once someone is diagnosed and needs rehabilitation, she said, but it should be used earlier to prevent health problems and reduce the impact of disease on quality of life. Cathy Maxwell added that there is a need for more education so that adults understand the processes their bodies go through as they age and can take the proper steps to take care of their health. While most people know they should not smoke or be sedentary, they need a better understanding of why these behaviors lead to poor health and how they can make a change for healthier aging.

5

Making It Happen with Implementation Science

Key Messages Made by Presenters

- Adopting an implementation science strategy requires identifying the contextual factors that either facilitate or challenge improvement of outcomes as well as the strategies that could be used to take advantage the facilitators and address the challenges. (Binagwaho)
- Health professions education should rest on sound educational strategies and pedagogies, and implementation science can be used to ensure that evidence-based approaches are effectively implemented into educational strategies, considering the local context as well as facilitators and barriers to change. (Thomas)
- Although the results of the service-learning study were encouraging, what was absent was the use of an explicit implementation science lens from the beginning. (Douglas)

This workshop, said Zohray Talib, the senior associate dean of academic affairs at the California University of Science and Medicine, has brought the concept of design thinking into the space of health professions education. During this workshop, she continued, speakers and attendees have heard from older adults about their lives and their needs, have identified a mismatch between the care needs of older adults and the health care workforce that will serve them, and have explored a number of "fantastic examples" of innovative programs and models that are making a difference. The next step, she said, is to take these best practices and expand, scale, and adapt them in new contexts. Doing this successfully will require using implementation science.

In this session of the workshop, speakers described implementation science and how it can be used to promote the uptake of evidence-based practices to improve health professions education and training and, in turn, improve and strengthen the workforce to care for older adults.

THE IMPORTANCE OF IMPLEMENTATION SCIENCE

The process of translating research findings into health outcomes is not automatic, said Agnes Binagwaho, a former vice chancellor and co-founder of the University of Global Health Equity, Partners in Health, Rwanda. Using the example of medical products, she said the process starts with basic science discoveries. Once promising evidence has been found, funds—usually private—are allocated toward the development and manufacture of medical products that can improve health outcomes. However, if the products do not reach the population, health outcomes will not improve. For example, vaccines were quickly developed in response to the COVID-19 crisis, but vaccination rates are low in many parts of the world. In most areas, the well-educated and higher-income populations are more likely to be vaccinated, and those most vulnerable—including the elderly and health professionals—were not prioritized. In addition, thousands of vaccine doses expired in developed countries while people in developing countries could not access them. Implementation science is critical for making sure that research discoveries reach the intended target and have a positive impact, she said.

Binagwaho gave a formal definition of implementation research: "Implementation research is defined as the scientific study of the use of strategies to adopt and integrate evidence-based health interventions into clinical and community settings to improve individual outcomes and benefit population health."[1] There are various frameworks to describe implementation science, she said; the framework in Figure 5-1 describes it as taking place in five phases.

The first step is exploration, she said; in this phase, stakeholders explore the contextual factors and the problem at hand. The second phase, preparation, involves selecting evidence-based interventions that are appropriate for the local context. Collaboration with different stakeholders is essential to ensure a realistic approach as, Binagwaho said, no sector can solve the problem alone. In the third step, implementation, a strategy is selected to ensure coverage of the intervention. The adaptation phase requires monitoring and evaluation to understand when, how, and why to adapt the intervention and the strategy in order to get the expected results. Finally, in the sustainment phase, stakeholders decide how to ensure

---

[1] https://grants.nih.gov/grants/guide/pa-files/PAR-19-274.html (accessed March 7, 2022).

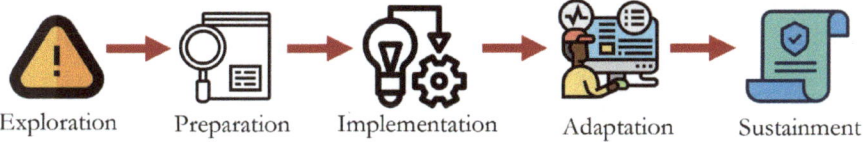

FIGURE 5-1 Implementation science framework.
SOURCE: Binagwaho presentation, November 17, 2022.

long-term implementation and sustainable outcomes through integrating the intervention into systems and policies.

Adopting an implementation science strategy requires identifying the contextual factors that either facilitate or challenge the improvement of outcomes as well as the strategies that could be used to take advantage of the facilitators and address the challenges. Taking the example of emerging health needs in an aging population, Binagwaho said that one challenging contextual factor is that longer lifespans decrease the incidence of deaths from communicable, maternal, neonatal, and nutritional diseases while increasing the incidence of deaths from non-communicable diseases. Strategies to address this challenge could include health awareness and prevention programs as well as long-term and end-of-life care. An implementation science approach also identifies facilitating contextual factors, Binagwaho said. For example, there is a strong community health worker program in Rwanda; strategies to take advantage of this strength could include having these workers conduct follow-ups for patients with chronic diseases or distributing drugs at the community level.

Once an intervention is implemented, its success must be evaluated across various dimensions. Binagwaho adapted Proctor et al.'s (2011) proposed implementation outcomes list to include:

- Appropriateness
- Acceptability
- Cost-effectiveness
- Coverage
- Effectiveness
- Equity
- Feasibility
- Fidelity
- Sustainability

She further emphasized that it is important to evaluate these outcomes in relation to each other. For example, a program that is cost-effective could be highly inequitable.

There is a need to build implementation science capacity at all levels of the health system, Binagwaho said. A country with a health workforce that is capable of doing research and implementing known evidence-based interventions will have a strong health system and will be ready to respond to new challenges, including the health needs of an aging population. Stakeholders who should be knowledgeable about implementation science include health care workers, systems managers, policy makers, and researchers. There is a strong economic argument for building implementation science capacity, she said: building capacity facilitates the use of all known evidence-based interventions and implementation strategies. This is key, she said, in strengthening health systems and ultimately contributes to economic development. In addition, there is a cyclical relationship between economic development, poverty reduction, and health. As the population becomes healthier, the production capacity of the country increases, which in turn promotes economic development and poverty reduction, leading to improved health.

THE ROLE OF IMPLEMENTATION SCIENCE IN HEALTH PROFESSIONS EDUCATION

Aliki Thomas, an associate professor at the School of Physical and Occupational Therapy and an associate member of the Institute of Health Sciences Education, Faculty of Medicine and Health Sciences, McGill University, shared her perspective on implementation science and how it can be used to improve health professions education. Thomas described the process of translating research into practice as occurring in three phases (Figure 5-2). Phase 1 involves identifying the nature and the magnitude of the research–practice gap; that is, to what extent do current educational practices vary from best practices supported by evidence? Phase 2 identifies factors that support or inhibit the use of evidence to inform practice; these factors may be at the individual, organizational, or systems level. For example, individual factors could be attitudes towards best practices or the skills to offer them; organizational factors could be the resources available to implement best practices; and systems factors could be accreditation standards that either facilitate or present a barrier to evidence-based educational practice. In Phase 3, interventions to reduce the research-practice gap are designed, implemented, and evaluated. In this step, Thomas said, it is critical to consider a number of questions:

- What do you want your intervention to achieve and for whom?
- What constitutes the intervention?
- How do you propose the intervention will work?
- How will you deliver the intervention?
- How will the intervention be evaluated? What does success look like?

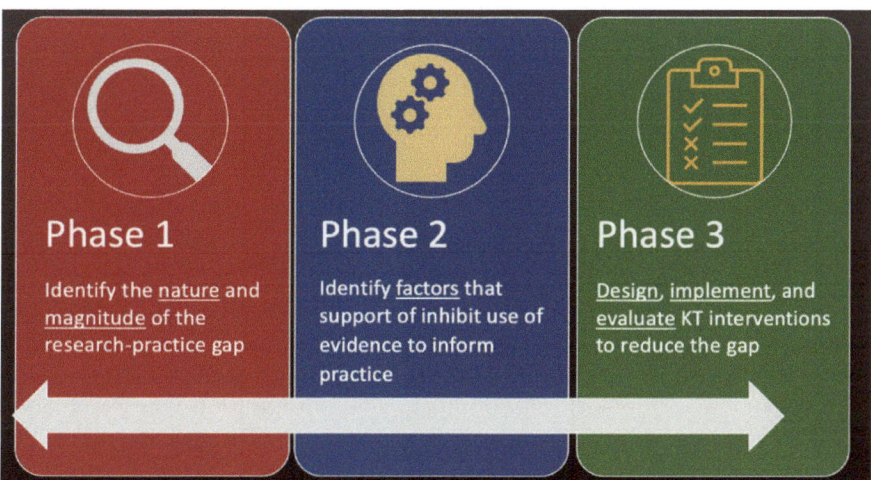

FIGURE 5-2 Moving evidence into educational practice and policy.
SOURCE: Thomas presentation, November 17, 2022.

Thomas described how implementation science could be applied specifically to the challenge of preparing the health professions workforce to meet the needs of an aging population. In Phase 1, the goal would be to document the current educational strategies used in health professions education and determine how these differ from what is recommended in the literature. This could be accomplished through examining accreditation reports, reviewing evidence on the learner outcomes of interest, and mapping current practices to the existing evidence on the specific educational strategy. Phase 2 would involve exploring the perceived facilitators and barriers in implementing a new educational strategy or pedagogy. Methods could include interviews, focus groups, or a survey of faculty; and the barriers and facilitators could include available resources, support from faculty or leadership, and community partnerships. Based on the first two steps, Phase 3 would involve designing interventions that take advantage of the facilitators and aim to overcome the barriers to the uptake of a new educational strategy. Designers could use frameworks such as the Consolidated Framework for Implementation Research (CFIR) to guide this process. In the particular area of preparing the workforce to care for older adults, the barriers to address would likely include learner attitudes, the confidence of the faculty to teach the topic, and having limited time or resources to support teachers in their efforts to prepare learners. There are multiple strategies to address these barriers, she said, including faculty development, webinars, and stories or testimonials of successful implementation projects.

Health professions education should rest on sound educational strategies and pedagogies, Thomas said, and implementation science can be used to ensure that evidence-based approaches are effectively implemented into educational strategies, considering the local context as well as facilitators and barriers to change.

CASE STUDY: SERVICE LEARNING AS PEDAGOGY FOR CHANGING ATTITUDES

In this session, Natalie Douglas, a faculty member of communication sciences and disorders at Central Michigan University, presented her work measuring the impact of a service-learning project on students' attitudes about working with older adults. This presentation was designed to frame the roundtable discussion taking place after Douglas' remarks, said Thomas, who moderated the session. Douglas began by saying that she has long thought about implementation science from a research lens but had not considered how implementation science could be used to support the education she provides to her students. This service-learning project, she said, was not conducted with an implementation science lens; she expressed her hope that by the end of the workshop session, participants could help identify ways that implementation science would improve the implementation and outcomes of the project.

As other speakers have noted, students often have prejudiced and stereotypical attitudes about working with older people, Douglas said. She shared a quote from an undergraduate student:

Before arriving [to the nursing home], I pretty much thought I was going to a mental hospital. I thought the residents were going to be these hollow husks of a person, and I was going there to entertain them for a bit.

Ageist attitudes like this, she said, may steer students in health care professions away from working with older adults. To improve student attitudes in this area, Douglas and her colleagues developed a service-learning approach that combined classroom instruction with real-world experiences. Research demonstrates that these types of real-world experiences, designed to expose students to older adults, can have a positive impact on their attitudes. In addition, service learning is designed to be mutually beneficial to both the learner and the community or individuals the learner is serving and to provide opportunities for critical reflection.

The aims of Douglas's study were to determine whether the attitudes of undergraduate students changed after a service-learning experience in which they engaged with older adults. Shifts in attitude were evaluated using the Dementia Attitudes Scale and reflective journal entries. The study was rooted in the AAA framework (Mahendra et al., 2013), Douglas said. The first A stands for awareness; the experience was designed to emphasize the acquisition of knowledge and self-reflection on gaps in knowledge. The second A is application; during preparatory training, Douglas and her colleagues sought to develop interactional skills with older adults as well as develop reflective skills that could improve clinical practices in general. The third A stands for advocacy or attitude; researchers were interested in exploring whether and how attitudes shifted as students underwent these experiences.

This project involved 145 undergraduate students across two midwestern universities. The students were all majoring in communication sciences and disorders, and 23 percent reported having previous experience working with adults with dementia. The mean age of participants was 21.5 years, and 141 of the participants were female. Over the course of a semester, students spent between 15 and 30 hours interacting with individuals living with dementia in long-term care environments. Students engaged in a variety of activities, including conversation, activities related to the individual's hobbies or interests, crafts, games, and sensory activities (e.g., holding a hand, combing hair). Students were trained in all of these activities prior to their interactions, including specific ways to communicate with patients with dementia, such as TimeSlips or using photos or gestures to communicate. Conducting the program required resources for classroom instruction, on-site coaching and support, partnerships with communities that wanted students to visit, and physical space for the students and older individuals to interact.

Douglas shared the results of the study. Students wrote journal entries over the course of the project, and the first, third, and fifth entries were coded for positive, negative, and neutral attitudes. As seen in Figure 5-3, the proportion of positive attitudes in journal entries increased as time went on, while the proportion of negative attitudes decreased. Results from the Dementia Attitudes Scale confirmed these attitude shifts, Douglas said.

In closing, Douglas again shared the earlier quote from a participating student, but this time included his final line:

Before arriving [to the nursing home], I pretty much thought I was going to a mental hospital. I thought the residents were going to be these hollow husks of a person, and I was going there to entertain them for a bit. ***I couldn't have been more wrong.***

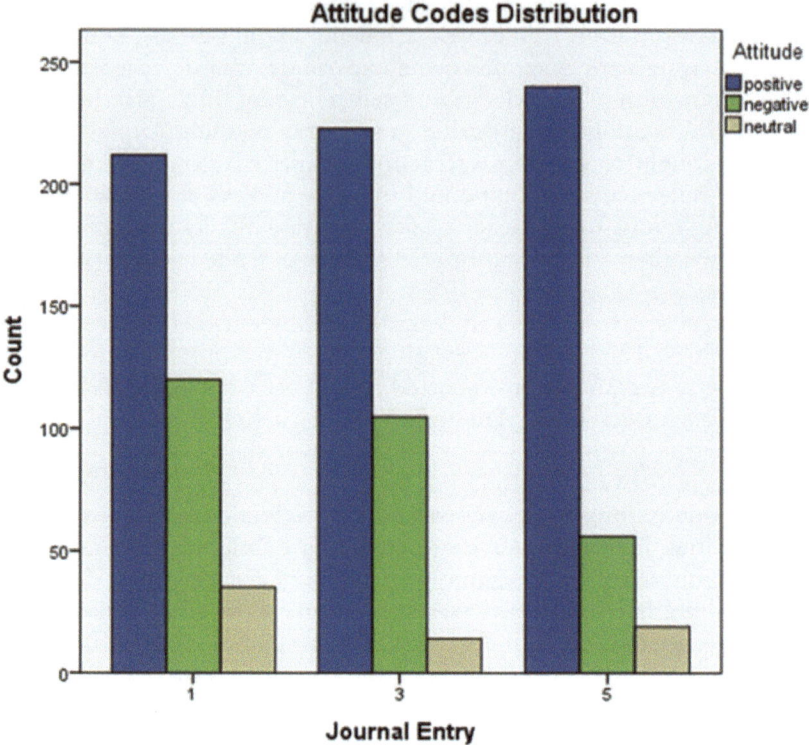

FIGURE 5-3 Distribution of positive, negative, and neutral attitude codes for journal entries one, three, and five.
SOURCE: Douglas presentation, November 17, 2022. Heuer et al. (2020), reprinted with permission.

Discussion

Although the results of the service-learning study were encouraging, Douglas said, what was absent was the use of an explicit implementation science lens from the beginning. Douglas and Thomas asked roundtable discussants to share their thoughts on using implementation science to systemically transform education, using both Douglas's study as well as their own experiences as examples. Each panelist was asked to describe his or her own experiences with service-learning projects and to describe the facilitators and barriers that they encountered when implementing these projects.

Thomas began by asking Douglas to use an implementation science lens and describe any facilitators or barriers that were identified when implementing the project. Douglas replied that there were a number of logistical barriers, including facility rules that required students to complete paperwork and medical testing before volunteering, finding the right point person in the care community, and finding times for visits that worked for both students and the care facility. An unexpected challenge, Douglas said, was the ethical difficulty of creating "beautiful relationships" that could only last for 15 weeks. A facilitator for both universities was the community engagement support each received from their institutions. The schools were applying for a community engagement classification, which created a high level of motivation to conduct this project. Another facilitator, Douglas said, was the relationships with the community care centers and the benefits that they saw from participating in the project. For example, some community care centers saw student participants as potential future employees.

Thomas asked other panelists to talk about their own projects and to describe the relevant facilitators and barriers. Toby Brooks, the assistant dean for faculty development at Texas Tech University Health Science within the Athletic Training Program, talked about his work in the graduate program on athletic training. Students in this program have the opportunity to work with patients across the age spectrum, and one challenge is educating the public and other health care professionals on their role in care. In recent years, he said, the program has focused on developing clinicians as educators and helping them acquire teaching skills at the same time as they acquire their clinical skills. Brooks divided facilitators and barriers into individual, organizational, and system-level determinants. Individual determinants include the formation and resilience of knowledge, skills, and abilities of individuals, and an individual and organizational determinant is the role of beliefs in the formation or development of practices. Brooks said that educating students with new knowledge and skills "doesn't do any good" if their underlying beliefs remain unchanged. An organizational determinant is the impact of program culture on accountability and outcomes, and systems-level determinants are the factors specific to the profession of athletic training (e.g., third-party reimbursement and the job market). Brooks said that the practices of implementation science are a useful way to see if health professions educators are "moving the needle" and making a difference.

Kim Dunleavy of the Department of Physical Therapy at the University of Florida, who was also representing the American Council of Academic Physical Therapy, said there are a number of different service-learning opportunities at her institution. These include interprofessional home visits, a community walking program, low-income housing chair exercise classes, balance and falls activities at a senior center, adaptive gymnastics, and a pro bono clinic. Some of these activities focus on older adults, while others do not; as a result, not all students gain experience engaging with this population. Dunleavy considered the question of whether the service-learning project model that Douglas described could be adapted for use in her community to improve learner attitudes toward working with older adults. Facilitators of this work would be the service-learning programs already in place, a number of existing classes related to the topic, and an established practice of encouraging reflective thinking in conjunction with service projects. Barriers might include the need for faculty supervision and faculty debriefing, challenges in integrating the model into existing coursework, and identifying a validated tool for capturing attitudes about working with older adults across the spectrum.

Dietitians work in a wide variety of settings and with a wide variety of populations, including many older adults, said Hannah Wilson, an assistant professor in the Department of Nutrition, Dietetics, and Exercise Science at Concordia College. At Concordia College, she said, it is a high priority to train students to be interested in working with this population and to be comfortable working in all types of settings. There are a variety of service-learning opportunities in both the undergraduate and graduate nutrition programs, including working with programs like Meals on Wheels. Facilitators of these kinds of opportunities, Wilson said, include a university-wide requirement for PEAKs (pivotal experiences in applied knowledge) and a graduate-level requirement for at least 1,200 supervised practice hours. There are also a number of barriers, she said, including a shortage of registered dieticians in older adult settings to serve as preceptors, a limited number of sites, the cost of testing and paperwork, and scheduling. The college has found creative solutions to overcome some of these barriers, such as using preceptors who are not dietitians and coordinating with nearby "competing" programs in order to find placements for all students.

CLOSING

In closing the workshop, Talib spoke on behalf of the Global Forum on Innovation in Health Professional Education's co-chairs and members, saying the challenge of building a strong health professions workforce to meet the needs of a growing aging population is not a distant possibility. "It is already upon us," he said, and it is time to use implementation science to take evidence-based approaches for strengthening the workforce and move them into day-to-day health professions education practice. Throughout this workshop, Talib said, he was reminded of a previous workshop that took a design thinking approach to explore stress and burnout in the health workforce. The idea was to bring design thinking—empathize, define, ideate, prototype and test—into the space of health professions education.

In reflecting upon that workshop, Talib said she believed that this workshop took a similar design thinking approach to the issues of educating learners and health professionals on caring for an aging population.

First, there was empathy. "We collectively brought a group of people together who are already naturally empathetic," she said. "But also, we heard the voices of our older adults and the learners themselves to really empathize with the issue." This is where the concept of design thinking begins, with the beneficiaries of our work front and center, she remarked. In the second part, the presenters defined quantitatively and qualitatively the status of the health workforce, the health system, and push and pull factors affecting the ability of health professionals to meet the needs of older adults. This led to then ideating and prototyping. "I think we've heard a great number of fantastic examples," Talib said, which demonstrated the challenges facing health professionals trying to meet the needs of an aging population. The final step of a design thinking model is to test, but an additional element could be to disseminate.

There are a lot of available resources, Talib observed, and now is the time to access those resources or prototypes already in use in the educational health system and apply implementation science to establish best practices for moving forward in training health professionals to address the needs of an aging population through health professions education. With that final thought, Talib thanked speakers, panelists, and workshop participants and adjourned the workshop.

A

References

AAMC (Association of American Medical Colleges). 2018. *2018 Physician specialty data report: Executive summary.* https://www.aamc.org/data-reports/workforce/data/2018-physician-specialty-data-report-executive-summary (accessed April 22, 2023).

AARP and National Alliance for Caregiving. 2020. *Caregiving in the United States 2020.* https://www.aarp.org/ppi/info-2020/caregiving-in-the-united-states.html.

Administration for Community Living. 2022. *Profile of Older Americans.* https://acl.gov/aging-and-disability-in-america/data-and-research/profile-older-americans (accessed April 22, 2023).

Alzheimer's Association. 2023 Alzheimer's Disease facts and figures. *Alzheimer's & Dementia* 19(4):1598–695. https://doi.org/https://doi.org/10.1002/alz.13016.

Arias, E., B. Bastian, J. Xu, and B. Tejada-Vera. 2021. *U.S. State Life Tables, 2018.* Hyattsville, MD: Center for Health Statistics. https://www.cdc.gov/nchs/data/nvsr/nvsr70/nvsr70-1-508.pdf.

Aronson, L. 2019. *Elderhood: Redefining aging, transforming medicine, reimagining life.* New York: Bloomsbury Publishing.

Ben-Ur, E. 2020. *The innovator's compass.* https://innovatorscompass.org (accessed April 22, 2023).

Cesari, M., I. Araujo de Carvalho, J. Amuthavalli Thiyagarajan, C. Cooper, F. C. Martin, J. Y. Reginster, B. Vellas, and J. R. Beard. 2018. Evidence for the domains supporting the construct of intrinsic capacity. *Journal of Gerontology, A: Biological Sciences and Medical Sciences* 73(12):1653–1660.

Chang, E. S., S. Kannoth, S. Levy, S.-Y. Wang, J. E. Lee, and B. R. Levy. 2020. Global reach of ageism on older persons' health: A systematic review. *PLOS ONE* 15(1):e0220857. https://doi.org/10.1371/journal.pone.0220857.

Crestani, C., V. Masotti, N. Corradi, M. L. Schirripa, and R. Cecchi. 2019. Suicide in the elderly: A 37-years retrospective study. *Acta Biomedica Atenei Parmensis* 90(1):68–76. https://doi.org/10.23750/abm.v90i1.6312.

Dawson, C. M. P., A. O. Abiola, A. M. Sullivan, A. W. Schwartz, and members of the GERI Team Research Group. 2022. You can't be what you can't see: A systematic website review of geriatrics online visibility at U.S. medical schools. *Journal of the American Geriatrics Society* 70(10):2996–3005.

Gerontological Society of America. 2023. *Age-Friendly University (AFU) global network*. https://www.geron.org/programs-services/education-center/age-friendly-university-afu-global-network (accessed June 7, 2023).

Franceschi, C., P. Garagnani, C. Morsiani, M. Conte, A. Santoro, A. Grignolio, D. Monti, M. Capri, and S. Salvioli. 2018. The continuum of aging and age-related diseases: Common mechanisms but different rates. *Frontiers in Medicine* 5:61.

Hebditch, M., S. Daley, J. Wright, G. Sherlock, J. Scott, and S. Banerjee. 2020. Preferences of nursing and medical students for working with older adults and people with dementia: A systematic review. *BMC Medical Education* 20(1):92.

Heuer, S., N. Douglas, T. Burney, and R. Willer. 2020. Service-learning with older adults in care communities: Measures of attitude shifts in undergraduate students. *Gerontology & Geriatrics Education* 41(2):186–199.

IHI (Institute for Healthcare Improvement). 2020. *Age-friendly health systems resources to practice age-friendly care*. https://www.ihi.org/Engage/Initiatives/Age-Friendly-Health-Systems/Pages/Resources.aspx (accessed January 18, 2023).

IOM (Institute of Medicine). 2008. *Retooling for an aging America: Building the health care workforce*. Washington, DC: The National Academies Press.

Jimenez, E. Y., J. M. Long, E. Lamers-Johnson, L. Woodcock, C. Bliss, J. Lee, J. Scott Parrott, R. K. Hand, K. Kelley, J. K. Abram, and A. Steiber. 2022. Academy of Nutrition and Dietetics Nutrition Research Network: Rationale and protocol for a study to validate the Academy of Nutrition and Dietetics/American Society for Parenteral and Enteral Nutrition consensus-derived diagnostic indicators for adult and pediatric malnutrition and to determine optimal registered dietitian nutritionist staffing in acute care hospital settings. *Journal of the Academy of Nutrition and Dietetics* 122(3):630–639.

Lortie, D. C. 1975. *Schoolteacher. A sociological study*. Chicago, IL: University of Chicago Press.

Mahendra, N., K. Fremont, and E. Dionne. 2013. Teaching future providers about dementia: The impact of service learning. *Seminars in Speech and Language* 34(1):5–17.

Maxwell, C., S. Miller, and D. Lee. 2022. Frailty-focused communication (FCOM) for older adults. *Innovation in Aging* 6(Suppl 1):221–222.

Miller, S., D. A. Lee, S. Muhimpundu, and C. A. Maxwell. 2022. Developing and pilot testing a frailty-focused education and communication training workshop. *PEC Innovation* 1:100013.

Mitchell, L., M. R. Frank, K. D. Harris, P. Sheridan Dodds, and C. M. Danforth. 2013. The geography of happiness: Connecting Twitter sentiment and expression, demographics, and objective characteristics of place. *PLOS ONE* 8(5):e64417. https://doi.org/10.1371/journal.pone.0064417.

Nash, R. J., and E. R. Ducharme. 1975. A sociologist looks at teachers: Careers, realities, and dreams. Review of Dan C. Lortie, *Schoolteacher. A sociological study*, Chicago, IL: University of Chicago Press, 1975. *Journal of Teacher Education* 26(4):360–363.

NHCGNE (National Hartford Center of Gerontological Nursing Excellence). 2019. Core competencies for gerontological nurse educators. https://www.nhcgne.org/core-competencies-for-gerontological-nursing-excellence (accessed on January 18, 2023).

O'Connor, M. L., and S. H. McFadden. 2010. Development and psychometric validation of the Dementia Attitudes Scale. *International Journal of Alzheimer's Disease* 2010:454218.

PHI. 2023. *Workforce Data Center.* https://www.phinational.org/policy-research/workforce-data-center/#tab=National+Data&states=01&var=Employment+Trends&natvar=Employment+Projections (accessed June 7, 2023).

Proctor, E., H. Silmere, R. Raghavan, P. Hovmand, G. Aarons, A. Bunger, R. Griffey, and M. Hensley. 2011. Outcomes for implementation research: Conceptual distinctions, measurement challenges, and research agenda. *Administration and Policy in Mental Health and Mental Health Services Research* 38(2):65–76. https://doi.org/10.1007/s10488-010-0319-7.

Roth, S. 2022. New US population study projects steep rise in cardiovascular diseases by 2060. https://www.acc.org/About-ACC/Press-Releases/2022/08/01/16/37/New-US-population-study-projects-steep-rise-in-cardiovascular-diseases-by-2060 (accessed April 22, 2023).

Rowe, J. W. 2021. The U.S. eldercare workforce is falling further behind. *Nature Aging* 1(4):327–329.

Siddiqui, M. J., C. S. Min, R. K. Verma, and S. Q. Jamshed. 2014. Role of complementary and alternative medicine in geriatric care: A mini review. *Pharmacognosy Reviews* 8(16):81–87.

Spetz, J., and N. Dudley. 2019. Consensus-based recommendations for an adequate workforce to care for people with serious illness. *Journal of the American Geriatrics Society* 67(S2):S392–S399.

Stubbe, D. E. 2020. Practicing cultural competence and cultural humility in the care of diverse patients. *FOCUS* 18(1):49-51. https://doi.org/10.1176/appi.focus.20190041.

U.S. Bureau of Labor Statistics. 2022. *Healthcare Occupations.* https://www.bls.gov/ooh/healthcare/home.htm (accessed June 2, 2023).

Vespa, J., L. Medina, and D. M. Armstrong. 2020. Demographic Turning Points for the United States: Population Projections for 2020 to 2060. *Current Population Reports* pp. 25–1144. Washington, DC: U.S. Census Bureau.

Wager, E., I. Telesford, P. Hughes-Cromwick, K. Amin, and C. Cox. 2023. *What impact has the coronavirus pandemic had on health employment?* Kaiser Family Foundation. https://www.healthsystemtracker.org/chart-collection/what-impact-has-the-coronavirus-pandemic-had-on-healthcare-employment/ (accessed April 22, 2023).

WHO (World Health Organization). 2017. *WHO Clinical Consortium on Healthy Ageing. Topic focus: Frailty and intrinsic capacity.* Geneva: World Health Organization.

WHO. 2021. *Global Campaign to Combat Ageism—Toolkit.* Geneva: World Health Organization. https://www.who.int/publications/m/item/global-campaign-to-combat-ageism-toolkit (accessed April 22, 2023).

WHO. 2022. *Ageing and Health.* https://www.who.int/news-room/fact-sheets/detail/ageing-and-health#:~:text=By%202050%2C%20the%20world's%20population,2050%20to%20reach%20426%20million (accessed June 2, 2023).

Zhou, Y., and L. Ma. 2022. Intrinsic capacity in older adults: Recent advances. *Aging and Disease* 13(2):353–359.

B

Members of the Global Forum on Innovation in Health Professional Education[1,2]

Patrick DeLeon, Ph.D., M.P.H., J.D. (*Cochair*)
Distinguished Professor of Uniformed Health Care Policy and Research
F. Edward Hebert School of Medicine and the Graduate School of Nursing
Uniformed Services University

Zohray Talib, M.D. (*Cochair*)
Chair, Department of Medical Education; Senior Associate Dean of
  Academic Affairs; Professor of Medical Education and Internal
  Medicine
California University of Science and Medicine, School of Medicine

Jonathan "Yoni" Amiel, M.D.
Interim Co-Vice Dean for Education
Senior Associate Dean for Curricular Affairs
Columbia Vagelos College of Physicians and Surgeons

Anthony R. Artino Jr., Ph.D.
Professor, Health and Human Function
George Washington University

---

[1] The National Academies of Sciences, Engineering, and Medicine's forums and roundtables do not issue, review, or approve individual documents. The responsibility for the published Proceedings of a Workshop rests with the workshop rapporteurs and the institution.

[2] Forum sponsors and in-kind donators identified in italics.

David Benton, R.G.N., Ph.D., FFNF, FRCN, FAAN
Chief Executive Officer
National Council of State Boards of Nursing

Agnes Binagwaho, M.D., M.(Ped.), Ph.D.
Vice Chancellor and Professor of the Practice of Global Health Delivery
University of Global Health Equity

Tanya Smith Brice
Vice President of Education
Council on Social Work Education

Reamer L. Bushardt, Pharm.D., PA-C, DFAAPA
Provost and Vice President for Academic Affairs
MGH Institute of Health Professions

Robert Cain, D.O.
Chief Executive Officer
American Association of Colleges of Osteopathic Medicine

Kathy Chappell, Ph.D., R.N., FNAP, FAAN
Senior Vice President
Certification/Measurement, Accreditation, and Institute for Credentialing
    Research
American Nurses Credentialing Center

Steven Chesbro, PT, D.P.T., Ed.D.
Vice President for Education
American Physical Therapy Association

Darla Spence Coffey, M.S.W., Ph.D.
President
Council on Social Work Education

Darrin D'Agostino, D.O., M.P.H., M.B.A.
Provost and Chief Academic Officer
Texas Tech University Health Sciences Center
American Association of Colleges of Osteopathic Medicine

Sanjay Desai, M.D.
Chief Academic Officer and Group Vice President of Medical Education
American Medical Association

Jan de Maeseneer, M.D., Ph.D., FRCGP (Hon.)
National Academy of Medicine Member
Department of Public Health and Primary Care,
Ghent University (Belgium)
Head WHO Collaborating Centre on Family Medicine and PHC—Ghent University

Kylie P. Dotson-Blake, Ph.D., NCC, LPC
President and Chief Executive Officer
NBCC, Inc., and Affiliates
National Board for Certified Counselors, Inc., and Affiliates

Kim Dunleavy, Ph.D., MOMT, PT, OCS
Associate Clinical Professor
Director, Professional Education and Community Engagement
Department of Physical Therapy
University of Florida
American Council of Academic Physical Therapy

Kathrin (Katie) Eliot, Ph.D., R.D.
Director
Health Professions Educator
The University of Oklahoma Health Sciences Center
Academy of Nutrition and Dietetics

Sara E. Fletcher, Ph.D.
Vice President and Chief Learning Officer
Physician Assistant Education Association

Elizabeth (Liza) Goldblatt, Ph.D., M.P.A./H.A.
Founding Board Member
Academic Collaborative for Integrative Health

Catherine L. Grus, Ph.D.
Deputy Executive Director for Education
American Psychological Association

Anita Gupta, D.O., Pharm.D., M.P.P.
Head, Chief, Comprehensive Pain Management
Scripps MD Anderson Cancer Center

Kendra Harrington, PT, D.P.T., M.S.
Board-Certified Clinical Specialist in Women's Health Physical Therapy
Director, Residency/Fellowship Accreditation
American Board of Physical Therapy Residency and Fellowship Education
American Physical Therapy Association

Neil Harvison, Ph.D., OTR/L, FAOTA
Chief Academic and Scientific Affairs Officer
American Occupational Therapy Association

Eric Holmboe, M.D.
Senior Vice President
Milestones Development and Evaluation
Accreditation Council for Graduate Medical Education

Lisa Howley, M.Ed., Ph.D.
Senior Director of Strategic Initiatives and Partnerships
Association of American Medical Colleges

Cheryl L. Hoying, Ph.D., R.N., NEA-BC, FAONL, FACHE, FAAN
Senior Consultant
Values Coach Inc.
National League for Nursing

Holly Humphrey, M.D.
President
Josiah Macy Jr. Foundation

Emilia Iwu, M.S.N., R.N., APNC, FWACN
Ph.D. Scholar
Rutgers University

Nasreen Jessani, D.P.H, Ms.P.H.
Associate Faculty
Johns Hopkins Bloomberg School of Public Health
Faculty: Senior Researcher
Stellenbosch University

Phyllis M. King, Ph.D., OT, FAOTA, FASAHP
Associate Vice Chancellor for Academic Affairs
University of Wisconsin-Milwaukee
Chair
Association of Schools Advancing Health Professions

APPENDIX B

Kathryn (Kathy) Kolasa, Ph.D., RDN, LDN
Professor Emeritus and Master Educator Department of Family
  Medicine–Nutrition and Patient Education
East Carolina University Brody School of Medicine
Academy of Nutrition and Dietetics

Albert Lee, M.D., M.P.H., FRCP
Professor (Clinical)
JC School of Public Health and Primary Care
Director
Centre for Health Education and Health Promotion
The Chinese University of Hong Kong

Kimberly Lomis, M.D.
Vice President for Undergraduate Medical Education Innovations
American Medical Association

Beverly Malone, Ph.D., R.N., FAAN
National Academy of Medicine Member
Chief Executive Officer
National League for Nursing

Mary E. (Beth) Mancini, R.N., Ph.D., N.E.-B.C., FAHA, ANEF, FAAN
Associate Dean and Chair, Undergraduate Nursing Programs
Baylor Professor for Healthcare Research
The University of Texas at Arlington
College of Nursing
Past President
Society for Simulation in Healthcare

Dawn M. Mancuso, MAM, CAE, FASAE
Executive Director
Association of Schools and Colleges of Optometry

Angelo McClain, Ph.D., LICSW
Chief Executive Officer
National Association of Social Workers

Lemmietta G. McNeilly, Ph.D., CCC-SLP, CAE
Chief Staff Officer, Speech-Language Pathology
ASHA Fellow
American Speech-Language-Hearing Association

Mark Merrick, Ph.D., ATC, FNATA
Professor and Dean
College of Health and Human Services
University of Toledo
Athletic Training Strategic Alliance

Suzanne Miyamoto, Ph.D., R.N., FAAN
Chief Executive Officer
American Academy of Nursing

Warren Newton, M.D., M.P.H.
President and Chief Executive Officer Elect
American Board of Family Medicine

Loretta Nunez, M.A., Au.D., CCC-A/SLP, FNAP
ASHA Fellow
Director of Academic Affairs and Research Education
American Speech-Language-Hearing Association

David O'Bryon, J.D., CAE
President
Association of Chiropractic Colleges
Immediate-Past Chair
Academic Collaborative for Integrative Health

Bjorg Palsdottir, M.P.A.
Executive Director and Cofounder
Training for Health Equity Network

Erin Patel, Psy.D., ABPP
Acting Chief of Health Professions Education
Veterans Health Administration

Andrea L. Pfeifle, Ed.D., PT, FNAP
Associate Vice President for Interprofessional Practice and Education
The Ohio State University and Wexner Medical Center
National Academies of Practice

Senthil Rajasekaran, M.D., MMHPE
Chief Academic Officer and Associate Dean, Academic Affairs at the Khalifa University
College of Medicine and Health Sciences in Abu Dhabi, United Arab Emirates

Rajata Rajatanavin, M.D., FAC
Minister of Public Health
Government of Thailand

Sabrina Salvant, Ed.D., M.P.H., OTR/L
Director of Accreditation
American Occupational Therapy Association

Stephen Schoenbaum, M.D., M.P.H.
Special Advisor to the President
Josiah Macy Jr. Foundation

Joanne G. Schwartzberg, M.D.
Scholar-in-Residence
Accreditation Council for Graduate Medical Education (ACGME)

Wendi Schweiger, Ph.D., NCC, LPC
Director, NBCC International Capacity Building
Foundation and Professional Services
National Board for Certified Counselors, Inc., and Affiliates

Javaid I. Sheikh, M.D., M.B.A.
Dean
Weill Cornell Medicine–Qatar

Carl J. Sheperis, Ph.D.
Dean, College of Education and Human Development
The Texas A&M University–San Antonio

Jeffrey Stewart, D.D.S, M.S.
Senior Vice President for Interprofessional and Global Collaboration
American Dental Education Association

Melissa Trego, D.O. Ph.D.
Dean
Salus University, Pennsylvania College of Optometry
Association of Schools and Colleges of Optometry

Carole Tucker, Ph.D., M.S.
Associate Professor in the College of Public Health and the College of Engineering
Temple University
American Council of Academic Physical Therapy

Richard Weisbarth, O.D., FAAO, FNAP
Vice President, Professional Affairs for CIBA Vision Corporation
Alcon
President
National Academies of Practice

Karen P. West, D.M.D., M.P.H.
President and Chief Executive Officer
American Dental Education Association

Alison J. Whelan, M.D.
Chief Medical Education Officer
Association of American Medical Colleges

Global Forum Staff

Patricia Cuff, M.P.H., M.S.
Forum Director and Senior Program Officer
Board on Global Health

Hannah Goodtree
Research Associate
Board on Global Health

Julie Pavlin, M.D., Ph.D., M.P.H.
Director
Board on Global Health

Emma Rooney
Senior Program Assistant
Board on Global Health

C

Workshop Agenda

NOVEMBER 15

2:00 p.m.   Welcome from the Co-Chairs
- **Donna Ferguson,** Mental health and wellness program manager, Department of the Army Criminal Investigations Command, Department of Defense
- **Andrea Pfeifle,** Associate vice president for Interprofessional Practice and Education, The Ohio State University and Wexner Medical Center

2:05 p.m.   **Framing the Conversation**
Relevance of Implementation Science in Health Professions Education
Agnes Binagwaho, Vice chancellor and co-founder of the University of Global Health Equity, Partners in Health, Rwanda

Learner Reluctance in Working with Older Adult Populations
Cathy A. Maxwell, Vanderbilt University School of Nursing

2:30 p.m. Working with an Older Population: Implementation Science for Studying Learner Attitudes
Moderator: Aliki Thomas, Faculty of Medicine and Health Sciences, McGill University
Speaker: Natalie F. Douglas, Communication Sciences and Disorders, Central Michigan University
Dr. Douglas presents her study: *Service-Learning with Older Adults in Care Communities: Measures of Attitude Shifts in Undergraduate Students*

Roundtable Discussion: There are multiple potential frameworks that could be used for applying implementation science to implement the study *Service-Learning with Older Adults in Care Communities: Measures of Attitude Shifts in Undergraduate Students* in different settings with different populations. The roundtable will explore two general questions that could apply to any of the frameworks.
Moderator: Aliki Thomas, Faculty of Medicine and Health Sciences, McGill University
Roundtable Discussants:
- Toby Brooks, Athletic Training Program, Texas Tech University Health Science
- Kim Dunleavy, Department of Physical Therapy, University of Florida; ACAPT Forum Rep.
- Hannah K. Wilson, Department of Nutrition, Dietetics, and Exercise Science, Concordia College
- Ewan Williams, Medical University of South Carolina

3:55 p.m. Closing

4:00 p.m. Adjourn

DECEMBER 7

3:00 p.m. Welcome from the Co-Chairs
- **Donna Ferguson**, Mental health and wellness program manager, Department of the Army Criminal Investigations Command, Department of Defense
- **Andrea Pfeifle**, Associate vice president for interprofessional practice and education, Ohio State University and Wexner Medical Center

A conversation with Willie Ann Burroughs and Nancy Cruz

3:20 p.m.	**Educating Learners on Aging Across the Life Course** **What Matters Most** **Caitrin Lynch**, Dean of faculty and professor of anthropology at Olin College of Engineering Joined by Peg Wihtol, community member, and Ian Eykamp and Zoie Leo, electrical and computer engineering majors, Olin College of Engineering Q&A
4:00 p.m.	**Working with Older Adults: Treatment/Care, Prevention, and Health Promotion** Objective: To understand the importance of a person's social, community, and cultural developmental factors impacting their health in later years requiring treatment/care while promoting health and prevention Moderator: Cathy Maxwell **Opening speaker:** Ricardo Custodio, University of Hawaii West O'ahu, Kalihi-Palama Health Center **Roundtable Discussion: WHO's Intrinsic Capacity** (p. 65) "The new vision of the World Health Organization for ageing was articulated in 2015 in the World report on ageing and health (2). This moved the organization from thinking about health in older age as the presence or absence of disease, and encouraged us instead to look more at an older person's functional ability (FA). It also strongly endorsed the need for countries not only to cater more effectively for the needs of older people but also to provide their health services and care in a more integrated way." See WHO, 2017: https://www.who.int/publications/i/item/WHO-FWC-ALC-17.2 The IC framework comprises cognition, mobility, psychological, vitality, and sensory functions. We added social, family, community, cultural, and spiritual factors. Is WHO's intrinsic capacity framework the right model? **Interprofessional Discussants:** • Elizabeth (Liza) Goldblatt, The Academy of Integrative Health • Kathryn M. Kolasa, East Carolina University, Brody School of Medicine • Senthil Rajasekaranm, Khalifa University College of Medicine and Health Sciences

Reflections from a Learner:
- Brooke Hazen, DNP student in adult geriatrics, Vanderbilt University

Respondents:
- Zohray Talib, California University of Science and Medicine
- Catherine Grus, American Psychological Association
- Nancy Kusmaul, University of Maryland School of Social Work

5:15 p.m.   Closing/Adjourn

DECEMBER 8

9:00 a.m.   Welcome Back from the Co-Chairs
- **Donna Ferguson,** Mental health and wellness program manager, Department of the Army Criminal Investigations Command, Department of Defense
- **Andrea Pfeifle,** Associate vice president for interprofessional practice and education, Ohio State University and Wexner Medical Center

9:05 a.m.

9:20 a.m.   **Supply and Demand**
Is the Health Workforce Prepared to Meet the Needs of an Aging Population?

Objective: To explore the demographics of an aging population and the makeup of the health workforce in education and practice and to consider how ageism and other push and pull factors draw people toward or away from working with older adult populations

Moderator: Greg Hartley, University of Miami Miller School of Medicine
Speaker: Rebecca George, M.D. Candidate, University of California Davis

Roundtable Discussion on Ageism: Push and Pull Factors
Facilitator: Greg Hartley, University of Miami Miller School of Medicine

Roundtable Discussants:
- Lauren Mazzurco, Eastern Virginia Medical School
- Ryan Bradley, Helfgott Research Institute, National University of Natural Medicine
- Rajean P. Moone, Center for Healthy Aging and Innovation, University of Minnesota
- Jeannine Lawrence, Department of Human Nutrition, University of Alabama
- Barbara Resnick, School of Nursing, University of Maryland

10:15 a.m. Break

10:30 a.m. Problem-Gap
How Do You Build an Interprofessional Program for Addressing the Needs of Older Adults?
Objective: To learn about programs educating learners interprofessionally on how to address the unique needs of older adults

Moderators: Andrea Pfeifle and Donna Ferguson, Co-Chair
Forum members and the first 50 non-member virtual participants will be automatically sent into breakout groups. Each group will engage in two discussions at 30 minutes per session. All others will remain in the main room.
Main Room:
Two Presentations:
- Integrating the 4 Ms: Age-Friendly Health Systems Framework in CVS MinuteClinics: Accessing Age-Friendly Health Education Tool
  - **Co-presenters:** Mary Dolansky, School of Nursing, Case Western Reserve University, and Ann Pohnert, lead director of clinical quality, CVS MinuteClinic
- Transforming Attitudes about Memory Loss: With Learners, Care Providers, and Communities
  - **Co-presenters:** Teresa McCarthy, Department of Family Medicine and Community Health, University of Minnesota, and Teresa M. Schicker, Minnesota Northstar GWEP, University of Minnesota

Breakout Groups:
1. Learners' Perspectives
   Led by Brooke Hazen, DNP student in adult geriatrics, Vanderbilt University, and facilitated by Nicole Anselme, student liaison to planning committee; Lily Brickman, student in food science and human nutrition, University of Maine; Rebecca George, M.D. candidate, University of California Davis
2. Engaging Intergenerational Learners Through Age-Friendly Universities
   Led by Brooke Hazen, DNP student in adult geriatrics, ed and facilitated by Rajean Moone, Center for Healthy Aging and Innovation, School of Public Health, University of Minnesota
3. Continuing Professional Development in Interdisciplinary Primary Care Settings
   Led by Josea Kramer, Geriatric Research, Education and Clinical Center, and facilitated by Jennifer Kim, Vanderbilt University School of Nursing
4. The Virtual Interprofessional (VIP) Consultation Clinic
   Led by Kristen Roof, University of North Florida, and facilitated by Kathryn M. Kolasa, East Carolina University, Brody School of Medicine

11:30 a.m. Closing

12:00 p.m. Adjourn

D

Planning Committee and Speaker Biographies

Donna Ferguson, Ph.D., M.A. (*Co-Chair*), possesses more than 22 years of broad, comprehensive experience bridging federal government service, academia, and the private sector. She is currently serving as the Department of the Army Criminal Investigations Command Mental Health and Wellness Program manager. Dr. Ferguson has served in other career-enhancing positions, including chief of the Behavioral Sciences Education and Training Division, chief of the Behavioral Analysis and Research Branch, licensed mental health professional, clinical supervisor, and adjunct professor at Webster University and Drury University within their leadership, education, and counseling programs. She is the Department of Defense (DOD) 2021 recipient of the Spirit of Hope Award, which is given to an individual or organization who epitomizes the values such as duty, honor, courage, loyalty, commitment, integrity, and selfless dedication and who significantly enhances the quality of life of military service members and their families serving around the world. Her portfolio includes trauma/transgenerational trauma, intimate partner violence, suicide prevention, sexual assault, grief and loss, diversity, equity, and inclusion, and curriculum development. As a specialist in her field, she has been a keynote speaker, lecturer, and trainer to the U.S. Congress, DOD military commands, colleges and universities, mental health organizations, law enforcement agencies, and civic organizations. She is best known for her psychoeducational work titled A Tree called Trauma, teaching mental health professionals and clients how to understand trauma in order to correct its impacts. Dr. Ferguson currently holds a Ph.D. in counselor education and supervision; an M.A. in mental health counseling, human resource management, and human resource development; and a B.S. in psychology.

Andrea Pfeifle, Ed.D., PT, FNAP (*Co-Chair*), is the associate vice president for interprofessional practice and education (IPE) at Ohio State University. Dr. Pfeifle works with each health science college to further develop and implement a new curriculum for IPE, and creates new educational models of practice across the Wexner Medical Center to create a learning environment that best prepares students for the future of team-based care. Dr. Pfeifle comes from the Indiana University Interprofessional Practice and Education Center, where she served as its executive director for the past 6 years. She has an impressive and extensive career in education, having worked to advance interprofessional education and teaching collaborative practice models across medical and health science education programs for more than 25 years. In addition to directing the Interprofessional Practice and Education Center, Dr. Pfeifle was associate dean of interprofessional health education and practice and associate professor of family medicine at Indiana University School of Medicine and adjunct associate professor of physical therapy at Indiana University–Purdue University School of Health and Human Sciences. As associate vice chancellor for IPE at Ohio State, Dr. Pfeifle works with each health science college to further develop and implement a new curriculum for IPE and creates new educational models of practice across the Wexner Medical Center to create a learning environment that best prepares students for the future of team-based care. Prior to joining Indiana University, she worked at the University of Kentucky from 1998 to 2014 in various roles, including as instructor in the colleges of health professions and of medicine, as the director of education in the Department of Family and Community Medicine, as chair of the Interprofessional Education Working Group, and as inaugural director of the Center for Interprofessional Education, Research, and Practice. Dr. Pfeifle earned her doctor of instruction and administration, her master of science in instructional systems design, and a bachelor's degree in physical therapy from the University of Kentucky. She completed a postgraduate fellowship in media design and production from the University of Kentucky.

Riham Ahmed Abu Affan is a third-year medical student at Khalifa University in Abu Dhabi, United Arab Emirates.

Nicole Anselme, M.B.A., M.S.N., is a board-certified critical care registered nurse with 6 years of nursing experience in various specialties such as emergency, critical care, post-anesthesia, medicine/surgery, and school nursing. She completed a master of science in nursing in 2020 and is currently working towards completing an M.B.A. in health care administration. She possesses a strong passion for nurse innovation, design thinking, and strategy development to mitigate social determinants of health and improve population health in underserved communities. Her passion has been fostered through participation in hackathons and brainstorming events as well as by working towards developing an app to improve health literacy and patient outcomes. Her professional interests include research and scholarly writing, discussing topics currently affecting the nursing profession, and exploring opportunities to support changes in nursing practice and education. She enjoys mentoring students and newly licensed nurses and is a fierce advocate against nurse incivility and bullying.

Ryan Bradley, N.D., M.P.H., is a senior investigator and the director of research at the National University of Natural Medicine in Portland, Oregon, and an associate professor in the Herbert Wertheim School of Public Health and Human Longevity Science at the University of California San Diego in La Jolla. Dr. Bradley received his N.D. from Bastyr University in 2003 and his master of public health in epidemiology at the University of Washington in 2009. After completing a residency, Dr. Bradley completed 8 years of National Institutes of Health (NIH)–funded clinical research training, including 5 years in the Division of Cardiology at the University of Washington. He is the principal investigator or program director on three active NIH grants. In addition to his research and teaching activities, Dr. Bradley regularly presents on the intersection between public health and complementary and integrative health (CIH). In 2022 he was appointed as the licensed CIH representative to the board of governors of the Patient-Centered Outcomes Research Institute.

Lily Brickman, M.S., holds a master's degree in food science and human nutrition from the University of Maine, where she also completed her dietetic internship. She was awarded the 2021 Outstanding Dietetics Student award for the state of Maine in 2021. Her undergraduate honors thesis research, Identifying Cofactors Contributing to Food Insecurity in Elderly Maine Residents Living at Home, was selected for the Emerging Leaders in Nutrition Science Abstract Recognition Award Program from the American Society for Nutrition in 2022. Last week she successfully defended her master's thesis research, which also focused on geriatric nutrition and was titled Educating Dietetic Students on the Nutritional Concerns of Older Adults.

Toby Brooks, LAT, ATC, Ph.D., is a dreamer, a learner, and a doer. He currently serves as assistant dean for faculty development in the Texas Tech University Health Sciences Center (TTUHSC) School of Health Professions and as an associate professor and director of the master of athletic training program at TTUHSC in Lubbock. His masters and doctoral work in teaching and teacher education at the University of Arizona paved the way for a career as an educator, with two decades of experience in the classroom teaching athletic training, strength and conditioning, and general kinesiology coursework. He is a six-time recipient of the SGA Outstanding Faculty Award for the MAT Program and also received the Dean's Award for Excellence in Teaching in 2017.

Ricardo Custodio, M.D., M.P.H., is a farmer, pediatrician, and professor. He was born on Kwajalein in the Marshall Islands. Throughout his 40-year career he has provided health care to Hawaii's poor and vulnerable population living in Kalihi, Hilo, Pahoa, Kau, Waianae, Nanakuli, Kapolei, and Waipahu. He has overseen the design and build of multiple clinics and the implementation of many programs. This includes helping to start a health plan, a vaccine program, a medical school, a nurse practitioner residency, a health science division, and now a nursing program, all of them in underserved communities.

Mary Dolansky, Ph.D., RN, FAAN, is an associate professor at the Frances Payne Bolton School of Nursing, Case Western Reserve University (CWRU), and senior fellow in the Department of Veterans Affairs (VA) Quality Scholars program at the Louis Stokes Cleveland VA Medical Center. Dr. Dolansky is the director of the QSEN (Quality and Safety Education for Nurses) Institute. She has co-published two books on quality improvement education, co-authored several book chapters and articles, and was guest editor on a special quality improvement education issue in the journal *Quality Management in Health Care*. She has taught the interdisciplinary course Continual Improvement in Health Care at CWRU for the past 10 years and was chair of the quality and safety task force at the school of nursing that integrated quality and safety into the undergraduate and graduate nursing curriculum. She is co-director of the VA Transforming Primary Care Center of Excellence, which was instituted to implement and evaluate a longitudinal interdisciplinary curriculum for medical residents and nurse practitioner learners, and she is active on the CWRU Josiah Macy Jr. Foundation grant to implement interprofessional education for pre-licensure students in the health care professions.

Natalie F. Douglas, Ph.D., CCC-SLP, is a professor in the Department of Communication Sciences and Disorders at Central Michigan University. She has spent the last 20 years supporting people living with dementia, aphasia, and other communication disorders through clinical practice, quality improvement projects, teaching, and research. As a speech-language pathologist, she specializes in improving the ability to communicate one's feelings, preferences, and needs so as to support relationships. To this end, she is currently engaging in work related to pragmatic clinical trials and learning health systems.

Kim Dunleavy, Ph.D, MOMT, PT, OCS, FNAP, represents the American Council of Academic Physical Therapy on the National Academies of Science, Engineering and Medicine Global Forum on Innovation in Health Professions Education. She has extensive academic experience in physical therapy education at the University of Central Arkansas, Wayne State University, and the University of Florida. She is a clinical professor and the director of community engagement in the Department of Physical Therapy at the University of Florida. Dr. Dunleavy's training includes an entry-level professional physiotherapy bachelor's degree from the University of Cape Town, a masters in physical therapy from the University of Central Arkansas, and a Ph.D. in instructional technology from Wayne State University. She has been board certified by the American Physical Therapy Association as an orthopedic specialist since 1993 and was elected as a distinguished scholar and fellow of the National Academies of Practice Physical Therapy Academy in 2017. She served on the planning committee for the global forum workshop on the non-pharmacological management of pain in December 2018 and is on the planning committee for the 2022 workshop on exploring the use and application for implementation science in health professions education. She is one of two co-editors for a collaborative special edition on Exemplars and Models for Interprofessional Pain Education, a collaborative project initiated by global forum members and the International Society for the Study of Pain Education group.

Ian Eykamp is an electrical and computer engineering major at the Olin College of Engineering, and he is interested in potential careers in design and education. To him, design is the process of identifying the diverse stakeholders for a project and involving them directly in decision making to ensure that the project meets their stated and non-stated needs. He believes engineers should act not just as problem solvers but also as advocates for the people their work will serve.

Rebecca George is a fourth-year M.D. candidate and rural community health scholar from the University of California Davis School of Medicine. She has a 15-year background in consulting at the intersection of government, health care, and community. Her work addressed intersectional determinants of health in Medicare and Medicaid programming with organizations such as IBM Watson Health and the California Department of Health Care Services. For 8 years, she volunteered as an in-home care provider for people with life-limiting illness. Her longitudinal research on the correlation of county-level demographic diversity and increased access to palliative care resources will be presented at the annual assembly of the American Academy of Hospice and Palliative Medicine in March 2023. She is pursuing an M.D. to improve quality of life and health outcomes across the lifespan for people from systemically underserved communities, especially rural populations. As an aspiring family medicine and palliative care physician, she seeks to use education to empower people in shaping the story of their lives all the way up to the end.

Elizabeth (Liza) Goldblatt, Ph.D., M.P.A./H.A., is a founding board member of the Academic Collaborative for Integrative Health and Medicine (ACIH). She was the acting executive director for 3 years, the chair of the organization for 8 years, and vice-chair for 3 years. Dr. Goldblatt represents ACIH at the Global Forum on Innovations for Health Professional Education. She has been the official ACIH representative to the global forum for 12 years. She is the co-facilitator representing ACIH on the development of a national course that will support the advancement of interprofessional, collaborative, team based, patient-centered care in partnership with the Academic Consortium for Integrative Medicine and Health, the national organization that represents integrative medicine physicians, nurses and allied health professionals. She was a consultant on a recent Albert Einstein College of Medicine's Patient-Centered Outcomes Research Institute grant to study group acupuncture approaches for chronic pain. She was on the leadership team of the National Center for Integrative Primary Health leadership team, housed at the University of Arizona, that developed a collaborative on-line course in integrative health for primary health care professionals. She was on the initial curriculum development team of the Duke Leadership Program in Integrative Health. In addition, she developed the doctoral and master's degrees at the Oregon College of Oriental Medicine in Portland, where she was president for 15 years, has chaired multiple acupuncture/Oriental medicine accreditation site visits, co-founded two doctorate of acupuncture and Oriental medicine (DAOM) programs, and was a member of the American College of Traditional Chinese Medicine (ACTCM) doctoral faculty.

Dr. Goldblatt is a leading educator in integrative health and medicine. She has a master's degree in public administration/health administration (M.P.A./H.A.) from Portland State University in Oregon and earned her Ph.D. from the University of California Los Angeles.

She is currently an educational consultant focusing on interprofessional education and collaborative practice. From 2014 to 2017, she was the interim executive director for ACIH. She served as provost and vice president of academic affairs at the ACTCM from 2004 to 2014. From 1987 to 2003 Dr. Goldblatt was president of the Oregon College of Oriental Medicine (OCOM) in Portland. She served as president of the Council of Colleges of Acupuncture and Oriental Medicine (CCAOM), a national organization that represents over 50 colleges throughout the United States, from 1996 to 2002, was the CCAOM vice-president from 1990 to 1996, and was on the CCAOM executive committee through 2013. Goldblatt co-chaired the education committee of the North American Acupuncture and Oriental Medicine Council from 1994 to 2006. She served on the board of trustees for Pacific University, Forest Grove, Oregon, from 1994 to 2004.

Dr. Goldblatt has co-authored several articles and contributed to book chapters with a focus on integrative health, including the recently revised third edition of the *Clinicians and Educators Desk Reference* on complementary and integrative health and a recent National Academy of Medicine publication on organizational health and clinician well-being. She has presented at numerous national and international conferences on integrative health and medicine and served on several committees and nonprofit boards that promote access to health care, body/mind practices, and education. She is currently on the Academic Collaborative for Integrative Medicine board and on the Coastal Health Alliance board of directors at Point Reyes Station, California, and she is the treasurer of the Tibetan Nuns Project Board, an international organization that focuses on education and medical care for the Tibetan nun refugees in Northern India. In 2018, for the first time in history, she received the Geshe-ma degree from His Holiness the Dalai Lama; this degree is the equivalent of a Ph.D. in divinity.

Catherine L. Grus, Ph.D., is the chief education officer at the American Psychological Association (APA) and has been on the staff of the APA since 2005. She was named deputy executive director for education in 2010. In her role as chief education officer, she leads the association's efforts to promote psychology in education and education in psychology. Dr. Grus has played a lead role in the association's efforts related to advancing interprofessional education for psychology students, primary care psychology practice, the development of models and tools for competency assessment, and supervision. She serves as APA's representative to the National Academy of Medicine's Global Forum on Innovations in Health Professions Education, the Interprofessional Professionalism Collaborative, and the Federation of Associations of Schools of the Health Professions. Before coming to APA, Dr. Grus was an assistant professor in the department of pediatrics at the University of Miami School of Medicine, where she served as the director of an APA-accredited internship program. Dr. Grus is the recipient of many awards, including the Paul Nelson Award, the Friend of the Association of Directors of Psychology Training Clinics, and the Nova University Distinguished Alumni Achievement award. In 2016 she was inducted into the National Academies of Practice as a distinguished scholar and fellow.

Greg Hartley, PT, D.P.T., FNAP, FAPTA, is an associate professor of clinical physical therapy and medical education at the University of Miami Miller

School of Medicine and is currently the vice president (and immediate past-president) of the Academy of Geriatric Physical Therapy, a component of the American Physical Therapy Association (APTA). Dr. Hartley is a fellow of the American Physical Therapy Association and the National Academies of Practice. Dr. Hartley received a doctorate in physical therapy (D.P.T.) from the University of Miami in 2010, a M.S.P.T. (physical therapy) from the University of Miami in 1990, and a B.S. (psychology/biology) from the University of Alabama in 1987. He is co-author of two clinical practice guidelines for physical therapists, Physical Therapist Management of Patients with Suspected or Confirmed Osteoporosis (2022) and Management of Falls in Community-Dwelling Older Adults (2015). Dr. Hartley is the founding program director of the first APTA-accredited geriatric physical therapy residency, and he has served as both a board member and the chair of the American Board of Physical Therapy Residency and Fellowship Education. Clinically, he has practiced in home health, outpatient, sub-acute rehab, long-term care, acute care, and rehabilitation hospital settings. He has been an invited speaker for more than 130 national and regional presentations. Dr. Hartley's clinical and research interests are in geriatrics, interprofessional education/care, clinical reasoning, and physical therapist professional and post-professional education.

Brooke Hazen, M.S.N., APRN, AGPCNP-BC, is an adult-gerontology primary care nurse practitioner (AGPCNP) with a master of science in nursing (M.S.N.) from the Vanderbilt University School of Nursing (VUSN). As she was working toward her nurse practitioner degree, Ms. Hazen trained with the Vanderbilt Program for Interprofessional Learning to understand clinical care from a variety of perspectives. That training continues to deeply inform her practice and professional interest in geriatrics. Currently, Ms. Hazen is pursing the doctor of nursing practice (D.N.P.) degree at VUSN. Her professional practice has centered on health care for veterans of the U.S. military, who are predominantly members of an aging population. In addition to her clinical work with geriatrics, she is the president co-chair of the Middle Tennessee chapter for the Gerontological Advanced Practice Nurses Association. Throughout her career, Ms. Hazen has worked to understand the special needs of the aging population. Her goal in engaging with this workshop is to assist in global planning for a new generation of interprofessional health care providers who are well-equipped for the evidence-based care of aging people.

Jennifer L. Kim, D.N.P., is a professor of nursing at Vanderbilt University School of Nursing (VUSN). She is a certified gerontological nurse practitioner (GNP) who has coordinated older-adult health courses for VUSN nurse practitioner students since 2002. She is a graduate of the doctor of nursing practice program at New York University College of Nursing (2015) and of VUSN's master of science of nursing (M.S.N.) program (1997). She earned a bachelor of arts in sociology from the University of California Irvine in 1995. Dr. Kim works as a GNP in the long-term-care setting. She currently serves as the president-elect of the Gerontological Advanced Practice Nurses Association, and she was the founding president of the Gerontological Advanced Practice Nurses of Middle Tennessee. She is a Hartford Institute Primary Care for Older Adults Scholar (2012–2014) and Jonas Leadership Scholar (2012–2014). Dr. Kim was a certification exam writer for the inaugural APRN gerontological specialist certification exam by the Gerontology Nursing Certification Commission. She was an elected member of the National Hartford Center for Gerontological Nursing Excellence Expert Panel on Gerontological Nurse Educator Competencies and was recognized by the organization as a distinguished educator in gerontological nursing in 2018. Also in 2018, Dr. Kim was inducted as a fellow into the American Association of Nurse Practitioners. She is currently VUSN's principal investigator of the Middle Tennessee Geriatric Workforce Enhancement Program and recently received funding for a digital literacy program that will be provided for older adults in an underserved north Nashville community.

Kathryn M. Kolasa, Ph.D., RDN, LDN, is professor emeritus and affiliate faculty in the Department of Family Medicine and a professor of pediatrics at the Brody School of Medicine at East Carolina University. Dr. Kolasa earned her Ph.D. in food science from the University of Tennessee, Knoxville, in 1974. Her bachelor's degree is from the Michigan State University in home economics with communication arts. She served on the Michigan State University faculty from 1974 to 1983. At East Carolina University she served as chair of the Human Nutrition and Hospitality Management Department from 1983 to 1986. She then joined the Department of Family Medicine and has held a joint appointment in the Department of Pediatrics from 2003 to 2013. From 2004 to 2020 she served as consultant to Vidant Health, a nine-hospital system in eastern North Carolina. She was awarded a Kellogg National Leadership Fellowship in 1986. She has worked internationally in more than 20 countries. She has served as a consultant to universities (including accreditation and program reviews), government and nonprofit agencies, trade associations, and the food and pharmaceutical industries and as a grant reviewer. She served as an external advisor to the Children's Healthy Living program, a childhood obesity prevention program in the American Pacific (2011–2016).

In 2008 she received the Centennial Award for Excellence—Service from East Carolina University. She was named a master educator at The Brody School of Medicine at East Carolina University (ECU) and also received the ECU Board of Governors Distinguished Professor for Teaching

Award in 2002. In 2003 she began serving as a consultant to the Nutrition Initiative of the University Health Systems (now ECU Health). In 2004 she was appointed to Fit Families NC, a study committee for childhood overweight/obesity. She provided leadership for the development and implementation of the Pitt County Achieving Healthy Weight in Children Medical Nutrition Therapy Protocol, which has been adopted by pediatric practices throughout the country. Dr. Kolasa directed the Food Literacy Partners from 1998 to 2008. In 2001–2002 she played a leadership role in the preparation of the North Carolina Blueprint for Changing Policies and Environments in Support of Healthy Eating and was a member of the writing team for the three North Carolina plans to combat obesity. She has been writing a weekly nutrition column for the Daily Reflector in Greenville, North Carolina, since 1986. Dr. Kolasa is a licensed dietitian nutritionist (LDN) and a member of the Society for Nutrition Education, the American Society for Nutrition, and the Academy of Nutrition and Dietetics. She serves on many advisory committees. In retirement she is a volunteer affiliate faculty at the Brody School of Medicine, where she teaches nutrition to medical students and residents as well as mentors junior faculty in publication and presentation. She is a contributing editor for *Nutrition Today*.

Josea Kramer, Ph.D., is the associate director for education/evaluation of the geriatric research, education, and clinical center at the Department of Veterans Affairs (VA) Greater Los Angeles Healthcare System. She is the founder and director of the VA Geriatric Scholars Program, which is the national VA workforce enhancement program that integrates geriatrics into primary care practices. The Geriatric Scholars Program has provided tailored continuing professional development opportunities for the interprofessional primary care workforce since 2008. Components of the program have also been made available to Indian Health Service and tribal health programs, as well as a program developed for Indian Health Service public health nurses on addressing behavioral challenges with dementia. Dr. Kramer is also known for her earlier health services research on how the VA and Indian Health Service work together. She is an adjunct professor in the Division of Geriatric Medicine at the David Geffen School of Medicine at The University of California Los Angeles (UCLA) and an educator in the UCLA-VA Geriatric Workforce Enhancement Program, which is funded by the U.S. Department of Health and Human Services Health Services Resource Administration.

Nancy Kusmaul, Ph.D., LMSW, received her M.S.W. from the University of Michigan and her Ph.D. from the University at Buffalo School of Social Work. She is an associate professor in the baccalaureate social work program at the University of Maryland Baltimore County. Dr. Kusmaul worked in health care for more than a decade in nursing homes, hospitals, home care, and adult day care. Her research focuses on organizational culture, trauma-informed care, and the impact of trauma experiences on the workforce. She is particularly interested in the experience of direct care workers in organizations, particularly certified nursing assistants in long-term care settings. She is a member of the Baltimore County Elder Abuse Coalition and the Maryland Nursing Home Culture Change Coalition.

Jeannine Lawrence, Ph.D., RDN, is the senior associate dean and a nutrition professor in the College of Human Environmental Sciences at The University of Alabama. A registered dietitian, she teaches clinical nutrition and nutrition research methods to undergraduate and graduate nutrition students. Dr. Lawrence's research focuses on nutrition assessment and interventions with nutritionally at-risk populations, particularly older adults, and using interprofessional education to improve health care outcomes in these populations.

Zoie Leo is an undergraduate student at Olin College of Engineering, where she is studying mechanical engineering. She has a humanities concentration in studio art. She is from Worcester, Massachusetts.

Caitrin Lynch, M.A., Ph.D., has professional experience that includes an assistant professorship in anthropology at Drew University as well as several fellowships, including a Mellon Postdoctoral Fellowship at Johns Hopkins University. She has taught at the University of Chicago and the University of Illinois at Chicago and is currently a visiting research associate in the Department of Anthropology at Brandeis University. At the Olin College of Engineering she teaches in the arts, humanities, and social sciences program. She is the secretary of the American Ethnological Society (of the American Anthropological Association) and past treasurer of the American Institute of Sri Lankan Studies. She is the author of two books, *Retirement on the Line: Age, Work, and Value in An American Factory* and *Juki Girls, Good Girls: Gender and Cultural Politics in Sri Lanka's Global Garment Industry*. She is also producer of the documentary film *My Name is Julius*. Dr. Lynch received her Ph.D. and M.A. in cultural anthropology from the University of Chicago and her B.A. in anthropology from Bates College. Dr. Lynch's research and teaching passions include examining the dynamics of work and cultural values (with a focus on aging and gender) as well as the cultural dimensions of offshore manufacturing plus a commitment to understanding social behavior in global contexts and a devotion to encouraging students to use qualitative methods to think critically about the world around them. She especially strives to expose engineering students to critical analysis and identification of the needs and opportunities in our aging world. One outlet for these efforts is in her interdisciplinary service-learning course Engineering For Humanity: Helping Elders Age in Place through Partnerships for Healthy Living.

Cathy A. Maxwell, Ph.D., RN, FAAN, carries out research directed at understanding outcome trajectories of older adults related to functional decline and frailty. She received her B.S.N. and M.S.N. from Troy University and her Ph.D. from Vanderbilt University in 2012. After completing a 2-year postdoctoral fellowship, she assumed a faculty position at Vanderbilt University School of Nursing in 2014. Dr. Maxwell's research has centered around the concept of frailty. She has examined outcomes in relationship to older adults' frailty status and reported 1-year outcomes of older adults hospitalized for an injury (falls), including functional decline, re-admissions to acute care, and mortality. Dr. Maxwell is interested in empowering older adults to manage their personal trajectories of aging. She developed a frailty-focused communication aid and associated workshop to train health care professionals who work with older adults to engage in focused dialogue about proactive aging. Most recently, Dr. Maxwell developed an educational tool for older adults to facilitate their understanding of the concept of frailty and to encourage proactive management of their personal trajectories of aging. She is interested in interventions with a nursing focus that empower older adults to engage in behaviors that enhance well-being and improve quality of life. She has recently received faculty seed funding to develop a video series on "mitochondrial fitness" aimed at promoting lifestyle change in the second half of life to mitigate the development of chronic conditions (i.e., neurodegeneration) and eventual frailty.

Lauren Mazzurco, D.O., has been part of the Eastern Virginia Medical School (EVMS) community and faculty, serving as an assistant professor of medicine, since January 2015. Prior to joining EVMS, she completed an osteopathic internal medicine residency at Botsford Hospital in Farmington Hills, Michigan, and completed a 1-year clinical fellowship in geriatric medicine at the University of Michigan, Ann Arbor. This was followed by a Department of Veterans Affairs (VA) special fellowship in geriatric medicine at the VA Ann Arbor Health System. She then went on to complete a fellowship in hospice and palliative medicine also at the University of Michigan, Ann Arbor. Dr. Mazzurco practices in diverse settings, including an inpatient palliative care consult service and a skilled nursing facility where she supervises third- and fourth-year clerkship students, internal medicine and family medicine residents, and geriatric medicine fellows. Most recently she has transitioned into the position of associate program director for the geriatric medicine fellowship at EVMS. Dr. Mazzurco is the director for case-based learning at EVMS and has served as the co-principal investigator on the American Medical Association Accelerating Change in Medical Education Grant, which supports the integration of health system science, chronic disease prevention and management, and high-value care into the undergraduate medical curriculum.

Teresa McCarthy, M.D., M.S., is a geriatrician and associate professor of medicine in the department of family medicine at the University of Minnesota. She is a member of the Interprofessional Geriatrics Coordinating Council for the University of Minnesota Northstar Geriatric Work Force Enhancement Program. She teaches medical, dental, nursing, pharmacy, and therapy students and created an interprofessional education team to practice and learn within a teaching nursing home site. Her research interests include delirium, falls, and medical direction in long-term care. She is a member of the American Board of Post-Acute and Long-term Care Medicine.

Rajean Moone, Ph.D., is the faculty director for long-term care administration in the College of Continuing and Professional Studies at the University of Minnesota. He serves as the associate director of education for the Center for Healthy Aging and Innovation in the School of Public Health. Dr. Moone's experience includes working at the Minnesota state unit on aging and area agencies on aging and leading Training to Serve and the Minnesota Leadership Council on Aging. He is a member of the Governor's Council on an Age-Friendly Minnesota, the Minnesota Association of Geriatrics Inspired Clinicians Board, and the FamilyMeans Board. He is a fellow of the Gerontological Society of America, a lifetime member of the Minnesota Gerontological Society, a McNair Scholar, and a Congressional/Health and Aging Policy Fellow. Dr. Moone holds a Minnesota nursing home administrator's license.

Anne Pohnert, M.S.N., RN, FNP-BC, is the lead director of clinical quality at CVS MinuteClinic and lead director of clinical quality for a national convenient care group practice of 1,200 clinics with approximately 3,000 nurse practitioners and physician assistants in 35 states and the District of Columbia. Her responsibilities include leadership of the clinical quality program at MinuteClinic, including strategic planning and execution of the Joint Commission Survey process and preparation in all MinuteClinic locations; leadership of the National MinuteClinic Quality and Patient Safety Committee; facilitation of multiple national quality initiatives; oversight of clinical quality metric development, implementation, and communication; annual review and update of all clinical and infection control policies and procedures; sponsorship of national shared governance councils for clinical quality; leadership of the steering committee and quality review team for the MinuteClinic customer relationship management program;

and facilitation of the clinical practice support committee, with a focus on clinical quality improvement in all practice areas.

Senthil Rajasekaranm, M.D., MMHPE, is the chief academic officer and associate dean for academic affairs at the Khalifa University College of Medicine and Health Sciences in Abu Dhabi, United Arab Emirates. He received his M.D. from Moscow State University of Medicine and Dentistry and his postgraduate medical pharmacology (M.D.) from Sri Ramachandra Medical University in Chennai, India. His work experience spans countries that include India, Ireland, Cayman Islands, and the United States. He was on the staff as a faculty member at the National University of Ireland Galway in Ireland and served in Decanal roles at St. Matthew's University School of Medicine in Grand Cayman; Wayne State University School of Medicine in Detroit, Michigan; and Eastern Virginia Medical School in Norfolk, Virginia. In his prior roles he was instrumental in establishing Centers for Excellence in Medical Education and served as its founding director.

Dr. Rajasekaran has been recognized by honorary fellowships from the American College of Clinical Pharmacology and the Academy of Medical Educators in the United Kingdom. He has received multiple institutional and national awards for teaching excellence and is a winner of the 2017 Costs of Care and American Board of Internal Medicine Foundation Teaching Value Challenge. He has received multiple educational grants aimed at implementing educational innovations. His grant from the American Medical Association produced a handbook titled *Facilitating Medical Education Transitions. Along the Medical Education Continuum.* Dr. Rajasekaran was part of the 10-member working group convened by the World Health Organization that led to the most recent publication of the Global Competency Framework.

Dr. Rajasekaran has been involved in the LCME accreditation as a site team member, and in his medical school leadership roles he has led their respective accreditation efforts. His areas of medical education research include accreditation, evaluating educational innovations in the areas, and teaching and assessment. He serves as the deputy editor of the *Teaching and Learning in Medicine* journal and is active on multiple international medical education societies and organizations.

Barbara Resnick, Ph.D., CRNP, is a professor in the Department of Organizational Systems and Adult Health at the University of Maryland School of Nursing, co-directs the Adult/Gerontological Nurse Practitioner Program and the Biology and Behavior Across the Lifespan Research Center of Excellence, holds the Sonya Ziporkin Gershowitz Chair in Gerontology, and does clinical work at Roland Park Place. Her research program is focused on optimizing function and physical activity among older adults, facilitating healthy behaviors among older adults across all settings of care, exploring the effects of resilience and genetics on function and physical activity, and testing the dissemination and implementation of interventions in real-world settings. This work has been supported by the National Institutes of Health, the Agency for Health Care Quality, and foundations such as the Helen and Leonard Stulman Foundation and the Robert Wood Johnson Foundation. Dr. Resnick has over 200 published articles, numerous chapters in nursing and medical textbooks, and books on restorative care and resilience in older adults. She has held leadership positions in multiple organizations including the American Academy of Nurse Practitioners, the Gerontological Advanced Practice Nurses Association, the Society of Behavioral Medicine, the Omnicare Pharmacy and Therapeutics Advisory Board, the Gerontological Society of American, and the American Geriatrics Society. Currently she holds leadership positions on the following boards: Gerontological Advanced Practice Nurses Foundation, American Medical Directors Association Foundation, National Hartford Center for Gerontological Nursing Excellence, and Omnicare Pharmacy and Therapeutics Advisory Board. She is also the vice president elect of the Gerontological Society of America.

As both a clinician and academician, Dr. Resnick has received a number of honors, the most recent of which include a 2014 honorary doctor of science from State University of New York (SUNY) on behalf of the SUNY board of trustees; the 2015 Dennis W. Jahnigen Memorial Award from the American Geriatrics Society; a 2015 induction into the Sigma Theta Tau International Nurse Researcher Hall of Fame; and the 2015 University of Maryland Regents Award for Mentoring. In addition to her own publications, Dr. Resnick is actively engaged in helping others disseminate their research and clinical work. She has been the editor of the journal *Geriatric Nursing* since 2006, is the associate editor for the *Journal of Aging and Physical Activity*, *Translational Behavioral Medicine*, and the *Journal of the American Medical Directors Association*. She has presented on clinical as well as research related topics nationally and internationally.

Dr. Resnick has an extensive history working across disciplines in teaching, research, and practice settings. This translates into policy initiatives, and she works among interdisciplinary groups at the policy level. She was a member of the Assisted Living Workgroup; currently represents the American Geriatrics Society on the Eldercare Workforce Alliance; and has worked on focused initiatives relevant to care of older adults with the American Geriatrics Society, the American Medical Directors Association, the Gerontological Society of America, and the Society of Behavioral Medicine. She is well recognized for her expertise in multiple areas and has served on numerous technical expert panels addressing quality measures across all settings of care as well as those specific to nursing homes and programs such as the PACE program. Examples of involvement include serving on the technical expert panels for the development of measures that will be aligned with the IMPACT Act of 2014; revising the late-life loss in function quality indicators for the Centers for Medicare & Medicaid Services (served as chair); and developing the catheter-associated urinary tract infections prevention tool. She has worked with the Centers for Medicare & Medicaid Services on numerous initiatives related to the Minimum Data Set development and implementation and on the implementation of quality initiatives such as decreasing antipsychotic use in nursing homes and other settings of care.

Kristen Roof, Ph.D., is a registered dietitian and an associate professor in the Department of Nutrition and Dietetics at the University of North Florida. Her major research interests focus on program development and evaluation using virtual technology. One program is focused on interprofessional education and communication among the health care team. The second program is focused on virtual project-based mentoring in dietetics. (See: www.rdmentor.com.) She is an expert at using innovative technologies in the classroom and in practice. Dr. Hicks-Roof is an active researcher, having presented her research at over 50 invited and professional presentations and having over 50 published articles and media. Using cutting-edge technologies, she has worked on several projects to understand whole-grain knowledge and sensory perceptions.

Teresa Schicker, M.P.A., is the program manager of the Minnesota Northstar Geriatric Workforce Enhancement Program at the University of Minnesota. In previous roles she led a national network to conduct research in interprofessional education and collaborative practice in health care and was the administrative leader of the Minnesota training center for the national implementation of TeamSTEPPS. Ms. Schicker earned a master's degree in public affairs from the University of Minnesota Humphrey School focusing on public administration and health. Additionally, she obtained a graduate minor from the Center for Spirituality and Healing. Her professional interests include health equity, interprofessionalism, and integrative healing therapies.

Joanne G. Schwartzberg, M.D., is a scholar-in-residence at the Accreditation Council for Graduate Medical Education (ACGME), researching the experiences and well-being of physician residents throughout their training. Prior to joining the ACGME, Dr. Schwartzberg served as director of aging and community health with the American Medical Association, where he developed multiple national programs to educate practicing physicians, residents, and medical students in implementing the latest concepts and guidelines into everyday medical management. These programs reached from 10,000 to more than 30,000 physicians on such topics as post-acute care and care transitions, home and community-based care, health literacy, patient safety, medication reconciliation, disability access, and older driver safety, with up to 75 percent of attendees implementing practice changes as a result (as reported 3–6 months after training). Dr. Schwartzberg has also served as an expert advisor on many panels and committees for governmental agencies (Centers for Medicare and Medicaid Services, Centers for Disease Control and Prevention, Agency for Healthcare Research and Quality, Office of Disease Prevention and Health Promotion, Assistant Secretary for Planning and Evaluation, Health Resources and Services Adminstration, U.S. Food and Drug Administration, and National Highway Traffic Safety Administration) and private organizations (United States Pharmacopeia, ACGME, Association of American Medical Colleges, Institute of Medicine [now the National Academy of Medicine], National Committee for Quality Assurance, and the Joint Commission).

Zohray Talib, M.D., is the senior associate dean of academic affairs, chair of the Department of Medical Education, and a professor of medical education and medicine at the California University of Science and Medicine. Her experience spans the field of medical education and global health, with a particular focus on social accountability in health professions education. Dr. Talib is currently serving as the co-chair for the National Academy of Medicine's Global Forum on Innovations in Health Professional Education.

Dr. Talib has worked with medical education programs in the United States and across sub-Saharan Africa to bring best practices, especially into low-resource settings. Her particular areas of interest include community-based education and building a robust and diverse faculty workforce for institutions in underserved communities. Dr. Talib's research across 10 countries in Africa sheds light on the value of bringing learners into community-based health care settings. Her research also examines the burden of mental health and strategies to integrate mental health into primary care. She has visiting faculty appointments at Mbarara University in Uganda, Aga Khan University in Kenya, and the University of Global Health Equity in Rwanda.

Dr. Talib brings to the field of academic medicine and global health the perspective of being a primary care clinician, educator, and researcher. She is a licensed and practicing internal medicine primary care physician. She teaches clinical medicine, health policy, and health systems to medical students. Dr. Talib was previously at the George Washington University, where she was associate program director for the internal medicine program and a researcher with the Health Workforce Institute.

Dr. Talib has a deep commitment to caring for underserved communities. Dr. Talib has worked in Central Asia and East Africa on community-based cancer screening, management training, and clinical research training for academic faculty. She currently chairs a national board that provides social safety net services including a crisis line, mental health services, and community-based care for the elderly.

Dr. Talib received her bachelor of science in physical therapy from McGill University in Montreal and her M.D. from the University of Alberta in Edmonton, Canada. She completed her residency in internal medicine at the George Washington University Hospital. She is board-certified by the American Board of Internal Medicine and is a fellow of the American College of Physicians.

Aliki Thomas, Ph.D., OT (c), erg., is an assistant professor and research scientist at the Center for Medical Education, Faculty of Medicine, McGill University. Dr. Thomas's research is on education and knowledge translation. She is interested in the development and assessment of advanced clinical competencies including evidence-based practice, clinical reasoning, decision making, and the development of professional expertise. Her work spans three major areas of occupational therapy education and practice, from admissions to professional education (including curriculum design and assessment) and clinical practice. In addition to her research in education, she is involved in research on how to bridge the evidence-to-practice gap where she uses an educational psychology perspective to examine the use of theory in the design and delivery of effective knowledge translation interventions. She is also interested in the concept of scholarship of practice and the outcomes of clinical–researcher partnership on clinical practice.

Peg Wihtol, M.Ed., graduated from Cornell University, Class of 1968, and received a M.Ed. from Framingham State College in 1973. Her careers included teaching junior high science, being an entrepreneur, and managing medical billing and offices. In retirement, she has been active as a part-time employee, a full-time caregiver, and a community volunteer. She has lived in Natick, Massachusetts, for almost 50 years.

Ewan Williams, Ph.D, is a research associate in the Department of Health Sciences and Research at the Medical University of South Carolina. They completed their Ph.D. in kinesiology and exercise science at the University of Georgia's Mary Frances Early College of Education, their master's degree in physiotherapy at the University of Birmingham, and their masters of science in exercise physiology at the University of Exeter.

Hannah K. Wilson, Ph.D., RDN, LRD, joined Concordia College in fall 2021 as an assistant professor in the Department of Nutrition, Dietetics, and Exercise Science. Dr. Wilson is also a licensed, registered dietitian nutritionist and serves as the coordinator of the Combined Dietetic Internship and Master of Science in Nutrition Program. Dr. Wilson graduated summa cum laude with a bachelor of science in nutrition and food science, with an emphasis in dietetics and minor in chemistry, from Georgia Southern University. She then completed her Ph.D. in foods and nutrition and a dietetic internship in the Department of Nutritional Sciences at the University of Georgia in Athens, Georgia. She holds a certificate in obesity and weight management from the University of Georgia Graduate School. Dr. Wilson's research interests focus on the influence of lifestyle interventions and improvements in diet quality on chronic disease prevention. She teaches nutrition, life-cycle nutrition, community nutrition, management, medical nutrition therapy, clinical experience, advanced medical nutrition therapy, and applied dietetic practice.

Dr. Wilson is originally from Dublin, Georgia, and now lives in Fargo, North Dakota.